Praise for *BreatheYou_ _____alance: Writings about Yoga by Women*, Volume One

"*BreatheYourOMBalance: Writings about Yoga by Women* is an incredible collection of individual experiences that speak to the collective journey via the practice of yoga. These pages are full of all the feelings; the highest highs and the lowest lows. As one starts to reflect on their own practice, the feelings become tangible, they resonate, and we relate. Each piece reminds us why we step on the mat and why we take that breath."—SHAUNA HARRISON, PhD in Public Health, creator of the #SweatADay challenge, Under Armour® trainer

"*BreatheYourOMBalance* is a pleasure to read. A book of writings by women, about women, it shows our struggles, challenges, and many victories. Through a yoga community on social media, these women have connected—and found the courage to share deeply personal experiences in the form of nonfiction, fiction, and poetry. They go deep into those dark places that make all of us vulnerable—places most of us have visited before—and overcome things like fear, anxiety, and self-loathing with breath and movement, love of oneself, and the light within.

"I have anxiety, too, and through yoga I have learned to control it with my breath. There are a number of stories that are relatable to me. I felt connected to these women by reading their words, by feeling their fears, by experiencing their joy."—ROBIN MARTIN, 200-E-RYT in Yoga Medicine, @robinmartinyoga on Instagram

"I'll never forget when I first met S. Teague, or @saltlifepirateprincess on Instagram. Her account was intoxicating and one of the few places to see a community of almost all women supporting each other's yoga practices and challenges. I immediately felt welcomed, even as a male practitioner, right into their community. Salty, and her friends, created a space where many could grow, expand, try new things, and even fail together—judgment free. A day wouldn't go by when I didn't check out what their community was up to. Now, seeing this book, *BreatheYourOMBalance: Writings about Yoga by Women*, come together is just icing on the cake. It is a perfect representation of the community that she attracted since day one. The love. The support. The family. It's all here on these pages. It came together beautifully and is only a small representation of how powerful this community of women actually is."—HUNTER COOK, @hunterfitness on Instagram

BreatheYourOMBalance®
Writings about Yoga by Women

Volume One

Selected and introduced by
S. Teague

Series Editors
Kitty Madden and Shana Thornton

TO: Danette & Joyce
All my love!
Clarissa ☺

Thorncraft Publishing
Clarksville, Tennessee

ISBN-13: 978-0-9979687-0-5
ISBN-10: 0997968702

Cover Design by etcetera...
Cover photo by S. Teague, SaltH2O Photography

Library of Congress Control Number: 2016953726

Part Two of "The Giving Moments" by Karissa Becker first appeared in *Mantra Yoga + Health*, Issue 13, Summer 2016. Reprinted by permission of the Author.

Thorncraft Publishing
P.O. Box 31121
Clarksville, TN 37040
http://www.thorncraftpublishing.com
thorncraftpublishing@gmail.com

10 9 8 7 6 5 4 3 2 1

CONTENTS

FOREWARD
By Shana Thornton

Gasping to breathe causes panic. I try harder, and my face turns red. My abdomen feels pinched as if with a sharp pin. I hold my diaphragm with one hand and the other shoots out from me, into the open air, as if my hand could grasp the air and place it into my mouth, but it eludes me as I panic in my desire for it. I signal the cheerleading coach that I'm coming off the sidelines of the field. The crowd cheers during the high school football game, and some of the fans follow us as my dad carries me away from the field.

After we reach the ambulance, they put an oxygen mask around my face. They tell me not to try so hard. They say, "Relax," but I'm afraid. They say, "Your body knows how to breathe instinctively." They remind me that I am healthy, an athlete, and that I'm experiencing performance anxiety. The shame associated with the word anxiety provokes the shorter, sharp breaths. I feel the panic begin to squeeze me again, as if a boa constrictor has wound tighter up my spine. The EMT tells a story as a distraction. Listening to the story, my breathing regulates. I remove the oxygen mask. We're all quiet. "Looks like you recovered," the storyteller says.

Years would pass while I searched for answers to my breath, and why I often lost my ability to breathe during stressful situations. I found breathing techniques in a meditation practice that I cultivated first and a yoga practice that I developed later. I discovered that breath is the gateway to the sacred, as it gives us life. Meditation practice was similar to the distraction offered during story-telling, but the affirmations and visualizations of meditations were more consciously associated with my ability to regulate my breathing.

As I discovered writings by women on the internet who expressed similar struggles and discoveries through yoga, I wanted to create a book about yoga by women, and that desire became *BreatheYourOMBalance*. For Volume One, the contributors are women from a variety of backgrounds and yoga experiences. They write about everything from the discovery of yoga, to sharing the practice with their children, from healing their grief, to overcoming a divorce; and from the simplicity of feeling alive when we breathe, to the sacred depths of spiritual revelation during meditation. These poems and stories exemplify our best recoveries of self through yoga.

BreatheYourOMBalance
Writings about Yoga by Women

INTRODUCTION
By S. Teague

There are very few places that spark a feeling of comfort in my life besides the walls that make up my home, and to be honest, sometimes that wasn't even the case. Part of being an approval addict is feeling deprived of the things you want or like. You are stuck in the mode of impressing others and following the trends set by whoever might be the trend setter at the time. Yet, I always had pieces in my life that felt like home. I still have a sleeping bag that I got from Santa in kindergarten and the Winnie the Pooh that my aunt and uncle brought to the hospital the day I was born. I longed to be surrounded by the feeling of home. Maybe it was for security reasons or maybe again I was just chasing what everyone else had taught me to chase. You see, for me home was a place, not a feeling. My house was always just a house, never a home.

When I want something, I am very creative in making it happen, usually. If I want a new pair of shorts and am not patient enough to go shopping, I will make them. If I want to color my hair, I don't wait for an appointment; I will color it myself. Because of all of my expertise in getting approval, I became very good at being a chameleon and very good at instant gratification to keep up with the Joneses. This is exactly the skill that brought me to yoga.

I ran across crow pose on Pinterest one day. The jock in me was intrigued, and I had to try it, and then another pose, then another. I was addicted. I noticed on one post an Instagram handle. So I downloaded the app and created @saltlifepirateprincess. I checked out all the yoga hash tags and sort of figured out all of the challenges and their quirky names. Something clicked inside of me as I was looking at all of the different shapes everyone was making. Women were being nice to one another.

The next day, I decided to post my own shot. I was just in tree pose, standing on the dock in front my house. I edited it. Funnily enough it wasn't in black and white but full color. I tagged it and I am certain that I wasn't following the rules correctly. I participated in challenges and annoyed the host with my odd poses that had nothing to do with their challenges, but no one ever said anything. I received so much love. Women were rooting me on and telling me how cool my hair was and what a cool location for yoga shots. I was addicted. I was addicted to kind words coming from women.

As many of you can relate, I spent a ton of my life being talked about by the people pretending to be my friends, or women had always been a bit catty to me because I broke a lot of the rules when it comes to proper hair and makeup etiquette. But, not on Instagram. These women were kind, loving and accepting of exactly who I was. My addiction made a turn. I was very addicted to finding more of me, or maybe I was more willing to *show* people more of me. I started by putting some thoughts I had on various things as I posted my pictures. Again I found support and love. I received continual cheering to be me and love who I was. To do me and let the haters hate.

Instagram became my diary. No one in my "real life" knew that I had an Instagram account. It was just for me, a world where I could nurture my thoughts, a place where I could figure out my wants and needs, a place where I was always accepted and praised even in my craziest of moments. My creativity and my art stopped being something that made people uncomfortable, and people found themselves entwined in the things I was writing. I found a group of like-minded women. I discovered a huge group, an endless group of women, who wanted to be accepted for whatever reason, and not only wanted acceptance but love for being who they are.

Many of the women that I speak of are in these pages with me. Many of them are more than Instagram friends. We know about each other's lives. All of us are very different but we are all very much the same. We support one another in more ways than social media. In more ways than one, these women are the voices that I hear in my head now. Their positivity drowns out the negative. In one way or another, we have grown together in our journeys.

As I mentioned, I always longed for a place that I could just be me. Not a house but a home. I wanted a place where I wasn't always looking over my shoulder to see who was next to stab me in the back. I was looking for a place to find my breath, a place where I didn't have to look for my breath, a permanent residence of comfort. I found it.

I closed on my new home one year ago. I repainted, furnished it to my taste, and remodeled a couple of spaces to meet my wants and needs. It's bold and very minimal. It's warm but very organized. It's fun but a place where things get done. I invite you to my house-warming party. These pages are the art that fill the walls, these women are my honored guests, come inside and breathe with us. Welcome home.

BreatheYourOMBalance

OOO
out of ourselves
Poetry by Stephanie Lasher

The hurt, the pain, the confusion.
Sunken ships from our yesterdays.
Relics long forgotten.
Rubble that settled down into our depths long ago.
There they remain in the hidden place submerged,
calcified skeletons that haunt our hearts and heavy our bones.
Until the day we come to ourselves,
and accept our first breath of life.
The floodgates swing wide as the waters rush in,
stirring up the sediment.
And we finally begin to feel.
We feel.
We feel.
We feel.
At first shallowly,
a glimpse,
a fleeting pang in a forgotten place.
And we continue to breathe
and we continue to feel.
We stay with ourselves.
And slowly, with time
the deep seated shipwrecks
begin to stir.
Dredged up out of the mire,
to the surface,
escorted by a hurricane,

a twirling, a dance of elements.
The breath.
We connect to our mud
and free ourselves from the illusion of clarity.
We realize that the ships we previously sentenced to remain in our impenetrable
depths are still ours.
Up out of the black we call to them.
The past we once thought needed to remain hidden away becomes the wind that fills
our sails,
the riding of waves,
the surfing of breath.
The breath.
The coming back to ourselves.
The process.
The churning up of waters.
The return of our story.

The story is yours.
The breath is yours.

Lungs + Yoga
Nonfiction by Tracy M.G. Riggs

Breath is important.

My senior year of high school, I was diagnosed with asthma.
Even typing those lines now gives pause to my heart. Asthma?

Having consistently led an active life, this rocked my world. I
remember the exact stoplight in my hometown where my mom and I
paused on our journey home from the doctor and I burst into tears; it
was raining and we had stopped at one of the biggest intersections in
our town.

Chronic illness. These words resonated in my head. No one that I
knew of in my family had asthma. I was not sickly, I was not weak. I
just had completed winning a championship volleyball tournament
with only three members of my team present. I mountain-biked and
hiked all over the hills of my beautiful East Tennessee hometown. It
did explain the massive fits of coughing that ensued after running and
training for volleyball. But, I was not that kid you see in movies
gasping for breath at the slightest of stressors.

Breath is important.

From that moment on, breathing and attention to breathing became
massively central to my life.

Breath is important.

Whenever stress arose, I would hold my breath, rendering me
exhausted and worn at the end of my day. I had panic attacks in
college, leaving me breathless and lying on my dorm room floor. I have
been hospitalized, medicated, and hooked up to breathing machines.
One of those machines still resides in my home. My lung capacity is
almost twenty percent less than a non-asthmatic individual. I have
wreaked havoc on my system through the serious antibiotic and steroid

medications that have kept me alive. I have had to combat the negative effects of these medicines with constant attention to diet, exercise and lifestyle habits that promote healthy living.

Breath is important.

Enter yoga. In 2006, I tried yoga to calm myself after a rough patch in life. I loved the strength that I gained almost immediately from vinyasa, bikram and ashtanga styles of yoga. I loved that breath was mentioned in every class, connecting movement to breath.

Breath is important.

Then, meditation followed. For whatever reason, I was convinced that meditation was going to give me an asthma attack. Meditation scared me; the thought of being still and just breathing in and out truly led me to believe that I was going to panic and the world around me would explode. Or, I would explode leaving tiny bits of my lungs all around the yoga studio. In my yoga teacher training course, I am required to meditate daily and journal about it. I started small—five minutes at a time. Now, I have sat for over thirty minutes, and I meditate daily. No explosions so far.

Breath is important.

The introduction of pranayama caused me to burst into tears and elicited a panic attack. After spending a weekend workshop with author Richard Rosen I was able to conquer my fear. I truly was frightened that Rosen would make us do breathing exercises akin to holding my breath for six minutes and then proceed to tell me I was not good at it and I would not be able to teach yoga, ever. All of this was of course ridiculous and Rosen looked me in the eyes in class and told me there was nothing to fear in his comforting way. Being a soft-spoken, bigger guy who you kind of want to hug, I believed him.

Breath is important.

Today, I get on a yoga mat almost daily. I slow my breathing down to focus on the relationship of movement and breath when on my mat, using breath as a tool and not something to fear. Whenever stress arises, I breathe. I meditate almost daily. I practice pranayama weekly.

As a result, my last trip to my asthma doctor literally saw an increase in my lung capacity.

Breath is important.

Recently, after one of my meditation practices, I checked my breathing with a Peak Flow Meter, which is used to gauge lung capacity in asthmatics, and my breath burst out of my lungs and I achieved a reading of 100 points higher than I have ever received.

Breath is important.

I am going to credit all of this to the work done on and off the yoga mat. Yoga removes residue of truly every part of your life. It cleanses you, and it may even heal you, as vinyasa yoga teacher Sri K. Pattabhi Jois believed.

In a 1977 lecture that's often cited in yoga articles on the internet, Pattabhi Jois stated, "A regular practice of postures with regulated breathing can cure many diseases. In order to cure contagious diseases a doctor's help may be required, but not to cure chronic diseases. Chronic diseases can be healed by postures and breathing practices."

I can at least say that this is true with *my* breathing. Through the work of yoga, I have become aware of my body and my breath, taking into consideration the things that my body needs and the things that harm it. Through the *tapas* (in Sanskrit, it means "to burn" and is often translated as the heat of discipline, referencing yoga practice and self-discipline) of yoga, we learn to cultivate purity, as a diamond is formed from the heat of Earth. We dig deeply into our bodies, minds and souls through our yoga practice and this reveals the areas of our lives that need 'tweaking' in order to function better. Yoga provides the awareness to better our lives, and resultantly the lives around us. Through yoga I have learned to harness the power of breath that I so desperately needed to make asthma little more than an annoyance, like a wart.

Breath is important.

Why Do We?
Poetry by Tracy M.G. Riggs

Why do we hold our tongues?
Why do we hold our breath?
Why do we strain our lungs?
Why do we worry to death?

There is a better way, we know
And yet, we continue on this path.
We could free ourselves and grow.
Stop hurting ourselves with wrath.

Why do we hold our tongues?
Keeping how we feel inside?
We hide in fear as if clinging to ladder rungs,
Hoping to find a peace within which to abide.

Why do we hold our breath?
Letting illness and stress arise?
Not breathing leads to death,
Letting go and feeling opens our eyes.

Why do we strain our lungs?
Keeping screams locked away,
Writhing our breath while we are young,
Losing our identity and voices in dismay.

Why do we worry to death?
Trying to be something we are not,
We troll around while others waste their breath
Dismissing all that we have got.

Challenge thyself then, to let go.
Find your voice and unlock it inside.
There are others who your story must know
Giving them empathy in which to abide.

Inhale, Exhale
Nonfiction by Jessica Gibbs

~December 2013~

I unroll my yoga mat. I don't know what I expect. Magic, maybe? It seems like everyone who does yoga is magical. Pictures of floating, effortless bendiness with long quotes by famous people that I can't make sense of, but everyone seems to gush over these magical beings.

And, here I am. Married. Unhappy. Staring at a cheap, green yoga mat my mom bought me eight years ago.

"Humph," I grunt.

It doesn't seem so magical to me, but I step onto the mat anyway, feeling the plastic cells of cushion under my feet. All I can think about is the life I left. I would no longer be dancing daily, and there definitely would be no aerial classes in this small Midwestern town. All I have is this yoga mat.

I turn on the computer, listen to the instructor, and then twist myself as much as I can into every pose. I want to "get it." I need to nail the poses. Every aspect of my life feels wrong. I feel like I am underwater, running out of breath, and I have no idea which way is up.

"And now take a deep inhale as we prepare for savasana," the instructor says.

I skip *savasana* (final relaxation pose, also known as corpse pose), red-faced, dripping of sweat and huffing. I skip all those breaths, but I keep coming back day after day. This green rectangle becomes a safe haven of sorts—a place where I don't have to deal with the unhappiness of my life, and a place for me to struggle with poses instead of emotions.

~March 2014~

I still don't consider myself a yogi. I practice a few times a week, and I still skip savasana. I unroll my green mat to exercise. It's not yoga to me. I'm not a yogi. I don't balance in picture-worthy poses with quotes rich in meaning underneath like the pictures online, but I still need this practice. I've moved with my husband to this small town, and it's winter, but not the winter of fluffy, light, snow-filled walks under glowing street lights. This winter has wind chills causing frostbite in a mere ten minutes—the kind of winter that sets up camp in your bones and the chill lingers until spring, which I've heard doesn't truly bloom until May.

I think about this on my mat after practice. How alone and angry I feel. Why did I move here for him? And I burst into tears on the floor of an apartment that feels cold even with the thermostat at 76 degrees. My sobs come out in choked breaths and tears glisten on my mat. Once my chest stops shaking and my breathing slows, I look out the window at the walking path below. I watch a cyclist in the distance, pedaling in an arctic spandex suit and helmet, and he is swallowed by the glare of white in the distance. And then I see a family of four, bundled in woolen gloves and hats, smiling and laughing as the husband pushes the stroller and the wife holds the young boy's hand. I store this picture in my head thinking maybe I could live in that picture. Maybe that could be what I want. As I roll up my mat, a small voice enters my head and says, "No, it's not." But I put it away in the corner, much like my green mat. How can I be so selfish to this kind person I married? No, these thoughts need to remain silent.

The winter rolls on with its gray skies and blinding white. Over the months, I practice over and over again, until physically I cannot practice anymore and fall into an exhausted, dreamless sleep, sometimes on the floor. *Eka pada rajakapotasana* (one-legged king pigeon pose). *Urdhva dhanurasana* (upward facing bow pose). The Sanskrit names float through my head as I try to ignore the growing silence in my marriage. He works. I work. I practice as he eats dinner. He watches television while I eat dinner. I focus on gaining flexibility and strength. He focuses on building his business. I don't focus on my breath in my practice. I don't notice how shallow and rapid it becomes when he is around. I close my eyes and try to fly in *eka pada bakasana* (one-legged crane pose), even for a moment.

~January 2015~

"I want to go to counseling," I say.

He looks at me and says, "Okay, you set it up, and I'll go."

We are sitting on the couch at opposite ends. I'm staring out the window and he's lost in some television series. It is winter again, and the families, cyclists and runners are under the window, moving forward. All I can think is, *I'm trapped inside.* Tears fill my eyes, hot and stinging.

"Why are you crying again?" he says, frustration rolling off his words.

I run to the bathroom, shut the door, turn around and sink to the tiled floor. This room is the only one with any warmth, as it is so small and the heat has nowhere to go. He doesn't even come to this side of the apartment anymore. He sleeps in the spare bedroom, and I sleep in the master.

Each of us say hollow goodnights and "I love you," and it is this thought that makes the tears roll down my cheeks and silent sobs rack my chest. I know he will come apologize soon. And I will too, as this is our married routine. Then I will go back to my green mat and do more yoga, skip savasana and go to bed with bloodshot eyes, a headache, and swollen eyelids.

~Valentine's Day 2015~

I buy a mala for myself and the proceeds go to a children's hospital where a wrist mala will be donated to a child with cancer. I've started to crave more than the physical practice of yoga. I want to learn to meditate and watch my thoughts because I am lost in my marriage and have no idea who I am anymore. Counseling has started and each session leaves me exhausted as the three of us sift through the elephants in the room and old wounds fester under the surface. He wants kids. I don't. I want to move. He thinks I can be happy here if I try harder.

And so I read everything I can about divorce, self-love, self-help, and meditation. I do all the exercises the counselor tells me to do. I start a daily practice of looking in the mirror and saying five positive qualities about myself.

I decide to use my mala and start meditating. I take the green-stoned mala in my hand. I feel the wooden beads flick past my thumb and index finger as I repeat, "I am enough." One hundred and eight times. On my green mat. I inhale deeply and let out a shaky breath and go to bed, still in my yoga leggings and sports bra.

~March 2015~

My husband and I kiss each other on the lips.

"Thanks for watching the dogs," I say.

"You're welcome. Have a safe trip," he replies.

I leave in my car, packed with a suitcase and my green yoga mat and green mala, destined for a week-long road trip of visiting friends I've made over the past decade all along the east coast. I don't know what I'm looking for. Answers, maybe. I spend parts of days alone in the car, daydreaming about moving away and living alone. I unroll my green mat at each stop, taking time to unwind each day. Handstands. Backbends. Twists. Forward bends. I take time to breathe in and out, sometimes following my breath and sometimes just trying to make it through the practice without thinking. My husband never calls, and neither do I.

Toward the end of my trip, I meet a close friend for coffee at a shop on the Chattahoochee River. We sit outside with warm mugs, spring blossoming, and the sun shining down. I miss this city. I tell her everything, the words flooding out of me like water over the banks. She stares at me over her cup and listens. I feel weight lifting from me as I admit all the thoughts I won't allow myself to have.

"I'm unhappy. I don't know if I can stay. I don't want to give up."

And then I ask the question, "How do you let go of someone who has been your rock for five years?"

She doesn't have an answer but wraps her arms around me, and then I am alone. My cup is empty. The sun has moved behind the clouds. I find myself wandering down the steps to the river, hearing it roar over the sounds of birds up in the trees. I feel drawn to a clearing by an abandoned dead log. And as the sun comes through the tree branches above, I feel my heart break open like the feeling of a *hollowback pincha mayurasana* (feathered peacock pose) that I had practiced just prior to this trip. I see green tipping all the trees around me, and the ground shifts. My mind and thoughts shift, too. I sit on an empty swing and observe my thoughts. Breathe in, breathe out. Don't cry.

~June 2015~

Our 5th wedding anniversary. The conversation is stilted, yet we try to have fun. I try not to notice my husband watching the television at the restaurant throughout dinner. At the end of the night, I think, *Perhaps there is a chance. We had fun bowling. Maybe this can work.*

"Do you want to have sex?" he asks.

The blood drains from my face, and I feel a pit in my stomach. He sees the answer before I say the words.

"I've reached my breaking point. I can't do this anymore," he says as he walks to his bedroom, and I go to the bathroom floor on my side and cry into the tiles. He comes and apologizes, and we go to counseling for our fifth session two days later. He's silent the entire time, speaking only when the counselor directly asks a question.

I meditate. I work. I journal. I practice. I go to counseling. Alone. My green mat stays out. I cry. I repeat. And two weeks after our anniversary, I inhale and ask to have a "talk."

"Having kids is a deal breaker for you?" I ask him.

"Yeah, it is," he replies from the opposite end of the couch.

"Okay."

"So what are we going to do?"

I inhale. I exhale.

"I think we should get a divorce," I say.

"Me, too."

And for the first time in two years, we hug and mean it. My head rests on his chest, arms around his waist with his arms around me. I feel his heartbeat. The sound of a heartbeat has always been soothing to me, rhythmic like the ocean. Rhythmic like the breath. I feel his chest rise and fall.

And then we say good night and sleep in our separate rooms.

In the morning, I question it all. My eyes are swollen halfway shut from crying. He has gone to work, and I somehow have to pull myself together and go to work as well. I unroll my mat as the tears well up again and sink to the floor. I fold my trunk over my leg into pigeon. Inhale, exhale.

Inhale, exhale. Inhale, exhale. Switch sides. I run through Sun Salutations and follow my breath and my eyes dry. I find a stool and sit to meditate, but my mind feels aflutter. I can't keep track of the thoughts zipping by, so I concentrate on my breath. Inhale, exhale. Inhale. I follow it from the base of my ribs to the top of my sternum rising. Exhale. My shoulders release down, and I feel the weight of my hands on my legs, my feet on the floor. The guided meditation ends, and it is time for me to go to work.

~August 2015~

As I unpack my belongings in my new apartment, I realize I am about to start crying. I unroll my mat, fold myself into pigeon pose and sob, surrounded by twenty cardboard boxes and my mattress.

Inhale. Exhale. Follow the breath.

Once my breathing returns to normal, I open my eyes and stare at my green mat. It's worn, scratched in a few places and definitely does not smell like plastic anymore. I think about the triumphs of poses it has seen. The savasanas. The meltdowns. The fights. The tears. And even the end of a marriage.

As I rest there, I think about myself. I realize my practice has evolved from the physical, and it is no longer just on the mat. I am able to look in the mirror with love and in turn see love in the world. I have taken this practice, this thing called yoga, off the mat. I clutch my mala with my hand at my heart. I have opened myself to yoga, and in turn, yoga opened me to the possibility of myself.

I sit up to meditate and flick the beads of the mala between my fingers, whispering, "I am enough." Over and over again. 108 times. And this time, I believe it.

The Sum of Parts
Poetry by Chelsea Wise

Each day I bring my pieces to this space. I come bearing them as gifts and burdens. The weary, livened, young, old, raw, weeping, laughing, foolish, wise pieces. The mother, daughter, sister, lover, creator, destroyer arrives.

All that I have carried.
All that I have collected.
All I contain.

To this mat.

Inhale, everything enters.
Exhale, everything leaves.

The alchemy of weaving these pieces together begins again.
Each day. Each time.

The asana moves into me as water moves through sand, seeping into and around each particle.

My spirit stretches taut with my skin, over ribs and lungs; over heart and limbs.

Time bends with my spine.
Here in this place nothing escapes the witness of this movement.

The external threads itself to the internal.
Strength and weakness find equal balance in their purpose.

This practice where nothing becomes perfect.

Where my power is found in the shift of a gaze, and the scooping of a shoulder blade.

Breaking Free
Poetry by Ariel Bowlin

When my strength first emerged it was tentative,
like blades of grass pushing up through snow.

It became bolder as I worked to find balance.

My body gained focus as I struggled to mix strength and flexibility,
so I could transform into a dancer.

As my strength grew, I became more confident.

I built my core to be a firm foundation for legs lengthened by daily
practice,
allowing me to float like a firefly.

I started to see outside the box when my world turned upside down.

I searched for my center and found my breath to stand tall on my own
two hands and invert.

When I chose to defy gravity, I meant to disprove everyone who said I
could not.

If the skin that I'm in fits too tightly,
I just take a deep breath and expand.

My lungs fill, my shell breaks open, and I burst through the façade to
occupy new space.

I've shed so many skins that there should be nothing left except
newborn tissue unable to bear the lightest touch,

let alone the hard press of life.

Shoulders shaking and elbows raw,
I sway on my forearms and remind myself to breathe.

When I split open my legs and stretch them out,
the left foot still lingers in yesterday
and the right foot reaches toward tomorrow.

To make them even and find the stillness I seek, I must face the place
I am in today.

That scared girl is still a part of me,
but she is not who I will be forever.

Only in balance am I able to take flight and be free
to be the me
that I've always wanted to be.

River Stones: An Essay on Loss, Yoga and Healing
Nonfiction by Amy Renee Bell

Memories. Colorful memories. Vivid memories. Memories of rich spices in the air as we wandered through the *sucs* (local fairs) in Arabia; the smell of the elephant's tough skin as my feet dangled over its back; the sudden fanning out of a hoopoe's crest with the green grass of our front lawn as a backdrop; the way the sand blew off the top edge of a dune and into the blue sky behind it. So many memories. My life has been a fairy tale. A place of magic and love and epic adventures and rich views and ever intriguing scenery. Combine all this with family love as deep as the stars are distant, and you get a glimpse of how I feel about my formative years.

I feel as if the richness of my life has allowed for any negative memories to just fade away. My childhood feels and sounds like a dream world when I recount the seemingly fanciful stories, and yet every ounce of it was real. In addition to diverse experiences and exposure to many places in the world, I have been blessed my whole life to be surrounded by love. This love has given me confidence in all that I am.

I've pondered confidence a lot as an adult; how some people have it, some don't. I was given the gift of confidence by my family. My parents are the most adventurous people I know and my brother and I grew up knowing we could do or be anything we wanted, go anywhere we wanted, explore anything we wished to explore. We weren't just told this, we were shown, and because of their example I've never been one to shy away from something new out of fear; fear of the different, fear of the unknown, or fear of failure. My family gave me confidence. What a gift. I've always been able to believe in myself and my abilities and so I dive headfirst into new things with a thrill of possibility instead of hesitation.

Not everyone has the gift of a fairytale life. My sweet mother was drenched with a lack of love. Neglect, emptiness, and abuse filled her early years. At the age of nine, she knew she didn't want to be like any grownups she knew. She, unlike me, did not have a shred of happiness in her childhood, and she knew without a doubt that she was unwanted.

She tried to take her life once, when she was sixteen. She recounted this story to me, when I had ears old enough to hear it. Sitting on the edge of her bed, her room dark, with the bottle of pills in her hand, shaking, staring it down with eyes unblinking, and thinking momentarily about what she was about to do, she reached with her other hand to open the bottle and suddenly she could not proceed. She felt two sets of hands, tiny hands, one set on each arm, gripping her arms tightly and keeping her from moving. She was frozen, physically unable to move. She did not carry out her intentions. She never tried to take her life again, and she never forgot the little hands.

It was eight years later that my brother was born, and seven years after that that I came into the world. She firmly knew that ours were the hands that prevented her from taking her life so many years before. In that moment of desperation and sadness she felt somehow that two little people did, in fact, need her.

It took many years, but my mother finally experienced love. She and my dad found each other several years after she had run away from her early life. They interacted with such intense devotion and a love so deep and connected, it was tangible. And not just tangible to those who knew them, but tangible to outsiders looking in. Her gift to me, one she never had for herself until she met my father, was that I have always known I was wanted, important, necessary to someone, necessary to everyone in my little world. She impressed upon me that I was important to her before she even knew me—and even more so when she recognized my little hands.

My mother was filled, overflowing with love, for the rest of her life. All my life I remember the intense joy that my mom felt in being a wife and a mother. She used to whisper to me often that she had always wanted to be *my* mom. *Always*, she said, it's what she'd *always* wanted.

She broke free of everything negative in her first twenty years to start a journey of filling the next decades with love. My life is the result of this amazing woman's complete devotion to becoming better than what she had been shown. Because of her I have always been surrounded by intense love that has been so alive and growing right along with me. I was always given room to grow, expand, and try new things. I was encouraged always. I have been loved always.

Because of this example, when I searched for my own love to grow with someone, I wasn't going to stop until I found an equivalent to what my parents had. The man I found is more than I could have ever dreamed up. Perfect, no. But perfect for me, absolutely. He continues what my parents always allowed—for me to grow, expand, become something new. I am still encouraged always. To say I am lucky, blessed, fortunate, does not even begin to scratch the surface. I am immersed in love. We have had three children and I am as devoted to them as my mother was to me. And they tell me they love me bigger than the sky. So immensely blessed am I.

While my life indeed feels like a fairy tale, there of course have been trials all along the way as well. No life is without trial. But when trials have come I have had all these beautiful souls to guide me through. I have been surrounded, filled, buoyed by love pouring in from so many sources. And my memories have glittered with sand, spices, vibrant colors, and my mom. She is in every memory. Always there. My largest source of love and comfort, the water for any thirst my soul has had. The one I have always turned to.

So what do you do when your main water source feels as if it has been shut off?

One day, what seemed very suddenly, the water stopped flowing.

When I lost my mom I spent days, weeks, months, not wanting to get out of bed. I *did* get out of bed. But only out of necessity to others, especially my husband, the kindest, most supportive man I know, and my children, the people who can whisper to my soul. I tried to be happy for them, but sadness gripped me with cold metal chains and no amount of laughter or fun seemed able to penetrate me. I felt so lost. I knew my life was still a fairytale, and that all my memories were still there.

However, the main character in my fairy tale was gone. It hardly made sense. I tried to realize that sometimes a main character has to perish in order for growth of others to occur. But the sadness! Growth feels strangled, halted, when in the depths of such sadness. She was too young. I didn't have her long enough. I felt robbed, torn in half, devastated.

It took me a long time to stop only existing and begin living again. I feel like I've only just found living again. I began to find it slowly, with time, when I first rolled out my yoga mat. The first time back on my mat I simply sat, in an inconsolable posture, with my legs crossed in front of me, my overwhelmed hands facing upward on my knees. And I sobbed. I couldn't think or feel anything but the void left behind. The hole in my heart. I couldn't see anything but my loss.

My husband listened when I needed listening, held me when I needed holding, gave encouragement when I needed to hear everything would be okay. That *I* would be okay. He would tell me to go for a run, go to the gym, to put on music and roll out my mat. Begrudgingly, I would listen. With some consistency, I soon realized I always seemed to feel better afterward. Had I felt like my old normal self I would have known this, but finding a new normal can take quite a long time. I came to trust his thoughts for me because every time I did something physical, broke a sweat, did something hard, came to my mat, I'd feel a little lighter, a lift.

In doing hard physical things, I began to realize I could handle hard emotional things as well. These thoughts crept up on me as tears streamed down my face during long runs; they came often during workouts when I got angry at heavy weights in order to continue lifting them, but it wasn't until I came to my mat that they really settled into my bones and in my mind and stayed there.

My mat became the place where I could touch my thoughts. Hold them, instead of running away from them or getting angry at them. Where previously I only found confusion, sadness, and shock at the reality of it all, that my mom was gone…and pain, a physical ache that the sadness caused me, I slowly acquired the ability to dissect my thoughts and move with them. It began like the cracking of a shell that I was trapped inside of. It hurt, and I didn't feel strong enough to break the shell. Yet, as I forced myself to move from one posture to the next, it was like taking a thought from my head into my hands, turning it over, looking at it from all angles, looking at it up close, then from far away.

I found that I could then be okay with the thought. I could take the heavy thought, "she's gone" from my heart and cradle it in my arms, examine it, set it reverently on my mat with me and move with it. Removing some of the weight, for a time, gave me strength to break out of the shell of my sadness. It was slow, this process, but coming to my mat allowed me a space to collect these thoughts and sit with them, to move with them, and to let them be okay.

At first they seemed like jagged boulders, getting in my way, causing me to trip and stumble, lose my balance. Gradually, with my heavy thoughts on my mat instead of being in my head and heart, I felt freer to move. They slowly became more smooth and polished, like stones in a river. They were always there with me, but I was flowing, moving above them for awhile, looking at them in a new way. They no longer seemed to block my path, but gave me something to look at and ponder instead. I found I could even use them to help me find balance.

When my practice session would end, I would collect my stones and boulders and put them back where I held them. They would continue to weigh on me, and so I would come to my mat more often so I could set them down for awhile. Now, I have grown quite fond of seeing them there. I see them now as polished stones, of all colors, keeping my mat flat on the earth, keeping its corners from blowing in the wind. My mom would like this. We spent countless hours at the river together, or at the beach, looking for stones just like these. Sometimes we'd hike with empty backpacks just so we could collect beautiful rocks to bring home with us. I feel like these stones, in a way, are a gift from her to me.

Over time, thoughts of sadness have become thoughts of acceptance. After feeling so very lost for so long, to then, finally, find for myself a space where I can be with my thoughts has helped me heal immensely. After many months of this process, I finally feel that I can meditate on more than just the pain I feel. It began with removing the boulders. Then the tears would come. With tears, the pain fell out of me. I could let go of it for a time, let it pour outside of me instead of allowing it to fill me to the brim. Each different sadness, each terrifying thought about her absence, fell to my mat, moistening the boulders and stones on its way down.

It turns out stones are more beautiful when wet; the moisture brings out their color. And now, more often than not, by the time my practice comes to an end, and I can collect my beautiful river stones, the moisture having evaporated from them, I feel good. The stones have been weathered and are smaller now. I still carry them into my heart, but I feel differently about them now.

As I flow with my stones now, I hear my mom's voice the clearest and the loudest. It's similar to the feeling you have when you've participated in an intense yoga class and you're resting in child's pose, downward facing dog, or savasana, and the teacher comes along, ever so reverently, and touches you...your lower back, your feet, or your shoulders. The moment that physical connection is made you feel attached, grounded, and more whole; just from a simple touch.

Those same intense feelings come to me on my mat, in my moments of greatest struggle, or in my moments of rest, and it is like my sweet mama is sitting there, right next to me. In child's pose, she kneels next to me with her hand on my back. In downward facing dog, she helps ground me further into my pose. In savasana, she rubs my feet. In poses where I'm reaching outward or upward, she's reaching back to me. It seems that those heavy thoughts, the heavy stones I painfully held in my hands and examined in the beginning, the ones I allowed to rest on my mat, have become her.

My yoga and my mat have been integral parts in my healing process.

Now, my mat is a comfortable place—a place to find understanding. As I lie on my mat, a collection of stones of all different shapes and sizes surrounding me, I meditate. With my stones there, I am able to meditate and progress past the sadness. Most recently, I tried meditating on my *muladara* or root chakra. I felt very alone. My first thought of my roots was immediately my mom, and I felt lost again, as if the tree that was supposed to be next to me was now gone. I pictured myself as a tree standing all alone in a clearing. A weak, solitary tree with drooping branches and nothing else around it. I readjusted my mat, added a few stones to my collection, tenderly held others in my hands, turning them over trying to see something new. And eventually the picture changed.

Now, there is a mighty tree standing next to mine. The tree from which I have grown. The one who dropped the seed into fertile soil. The one who shaded me when my leaves were tender and young. The one whose deep roots brought water up from the soil's depths to where my short growing roots could reach and my thirst could be quenched.

This mighty tree did not disappear. She *still* stands right next to me. We stand by a flowing river full of beautiful stones, surrounded by other trees. My husband's tree is there, with beautiful vines tangled and tying our branches together so when the winds blow we sway together. There are three little saplings that we shade in the heat of summer and our roots bring water from the depths for their tender little roots to reach. My father's tree is there, right next to my mom's. Her tree does not have leaves anymore, but vines still creep up her trunk and tangle her branches with the branches of my father's tree. And when the winds blow the two still sway in unison, forever joined.

My brother's tree, and the tree of his wife, and the six little saplings they protect and watch over are there. There are many other trees, friends both new and old, loved ones, and acquaintances, who have given me strength to grow my roots a little deeper, grow my leaves a little greener, go for a new color in fall, or try a new dance during a rain storm. The picture I see now is like an aspen grove, or a thicket of scrub oak; roots intertwined, having grown near each other for so long. Our root system has become like one enormous organism, living, breathing, growing, keeping each other strong.

When a tree dies, it still stands. Its roots still stabilize it in the earth. It can still offer a home for creatures seeking refuge. It sways in the wind, gets wet in the rain, its boughs collect snow in the winter, it provides growing surface to moss and lichens, and stability for vines to climb into its branches. So while my branches still grow stronger, full of vibrant green leaves and maybe a few blossoms in the springtime; and while my leaves still change into brilliant colors and drift to the ground in the fall as I get ready for rest and new life again, new things to come, the mighty tree next to me also stands with roots still in the ground. And our branches rub when the wind blows. It fills me with the same rich feelings I knew as a child as the sandy humid wind blew through the date palms. Our trees get wet together when it rains, just as my mom and I did when she'd take me out to dance in the rains that came only once a year. Birds rest in our branches and sing to each other reminding me of late night conversations and laughter. This mighty tree is always right next to me, shading me with the same love that helped my branches grow.

Now, when I lie down in savasana, I lie with my river stones. I might never heal completely. I will never be the same. But I don't need to be the same. The stones will always be there. Many stones are polished and smooth, others still have jagged edges, not quite as far along in the process, but I see their beauty. They do not seem as heavy with their character and shape. I have grown to understand them, appreciate them, know them as extensions of me. Just like these stones, I get to be new, refined, reshaped. I sometimes still find new ones to lie beside me. Often they are delicately wet with dew which brings out their unique colors and lines. I lay among them with sounds of the river flowing somewhere nearby, birds conversing above me as they rest from flight and I hear the wind as it swirls through branches. It is love. Love is always there. I am warm and peaceful, forever blanketed in the shade of a mighty tree.

Testing Positive
Poetry by C.T. Kern

One day your heels reach the mat
in downward dog, your palms
flatten solid, your torso
tucks against your legs in a pike.
You have tested positive for
Pregnancy, two lines = two people
and the doping has begun
flooding your joints with that which
makes you unglued. In exchange
you can no longer breathe.
You are a table, a cat, a cow.
Your breasts become spherical, each
an encircled universe in a bag of skin
heavy with the idea of feeding.
Your stomach another universe
that calms to movement but awakens
in stillness: a fish-flutter, a ripple, later,
limbs fighting the state of calm.
At the end of class, when the time has come
for rest, you lie on your back.
Your chest constricts as if the weight
of this child will not be carried in your abdomen
but on your lungs, your heart. You cannot breathe
with the weight of it. Your teacher says,
Listen to your body.

The Giving Moments
Nonfiction by Karissa Becker

I breastfed for six years. It was such a huge part of my mothering life, and now it's coming to a close. Breastfeeding was originally why I coined myself "TheGivingMom." I nursed while pregnant, and then when Lilith was born and we tandem nursed, I could see myself as that tree, giving so much of myself and not pausing to consider whether it was best for me, only knowing that it was their happiness I hoped to foster. I'm grateful now to have my body back, but a bit like the tree, I wonder what I have left to give. I mean obviously I still have so much to give, but it's been such a strange feeling.... To have them be so much more independent of me.

My son continued to ask on and off until he was five, and I'm sure mostly because his sister who is two years younger was nursing all the time. But they are very different Little Oms, and I was shocked to notice Lilith self-weaning before she turned four. Shocked and grateful, that is. Yet every time I start to think that we are done, she will ask one more time.

It's been one of those long pauses, but the day my parents left, she came right up to me and asked if we could nurse. I reminded her that all my milk is gone now and asked if she was certain she still wanted to nurse, and she grinned sleepily and said, "It's ok! Can we still nurse, please?" so I decided yes, she was being so sweet, I told her we would have to lie down; I watched her little eyes flutter the way they used to every day while nursing, and she slowly drifted off to sleep. I kissed her. She is so big but she is still so tiny.

I think to myself about my yoga practice, about how we are all slowing down and regressing a little so we can heal and strengthen our bodies and move forward even more powerfully than before. Life is truly all a dance, sometimes we are taking the lead and sometimes we are following; it can feel like we are moving backward, even if in the same steps as before. The actuality is, we are circling and cycling and always blooming outward. When I mother my Little Oms with patience, it reminds me to mother myself with the same.

***

I was settling my little ones down for bed last night. We sleep on two queen beds that have been pushed together. It's one big, mostly happy, family bed. We usually sleep with Lilith on my right side and Jude on my left, which puts Jude between Mom and Dad and Lilith next to the wall. This used to be fine but Lilith recently realized she would also like to sleep next to her dad. So, they have to trade places. I told them they'd have to take turns every night because there wasn't any other "fair" option. The change upset Jude, and last night he was getting worked up about how this couldn't happen anymore and that he wouldn't be happy with the new arrangement.

He wasn't going to calm down and I said, "Okay, let's meditate. I can see you're out of control and we need to be in control to make good decisions." I sat up and said, "I'll do it with you."

He said, "I'm still going to be angry."

And, I said, "That's okay. Let's try anyway." We sat in bed and started breathing. I could see in the darkness as he put his hands on his knees and the crying seemed to subside.

I waited for a few breaths. I could feel my own self shift into compassion. I put my hand on his shoulder and said, "I know you're angry right now. You know what, though? There's a voice inside your head and it's telling you to be angry.... You don't have to listen."

I waited another breath.

Silence.

I said, "You could even replace the voice inside your head with a new mantra. You could say to yourself, 'I can be happy because I get to sleep next to my mom.'"

He had stopped crying and I waited for him to speak next. He looked down at the bed and slowly started to lie down. I wrapped him up in blankets and my arms and snuggled my face into his and kissed him.

Another bedtime saved by meditation.

Guided Meditations
Poetry by C.T. Kern

She did guided meditations.
It was the best part
of the hour, lying
arms open, melted to the floor
each limb heavier than it would be
for a whole week, even in sleep
lying there. She would read to us—
like that best part of second grade,
the chapter books after recess,
with our heads on our desks—
and we would visualize what we
were instructed to:
the gray industrial air leaving,
the fizzing green air entering
our lungs, remaking us.
We visualized islands and sands
and forgiving ourselves.
The blowers would kick on overhead
in the open, gym-roof ceiling,
and sometimes it was hard to hear.
And so it was that I pictured
the canyons she told us to:
two canyons, side by side.
then the canyons were swaying slightly
in the breeze. It was hard to picture,
these canyons, swaying.
And my friend, beside me, heard
"cantaloupes" and set them rolling
mysteriously beside each other.
The AC rumbled off
and it was candles—candles!
we were supposed to be thinking of,
their flames unsteady but strong,
side by side, each of us,
with our own small light.

The Morning Practice
Nonfiction by Regan Warner

My alarm rings, but I've been awake waiting for it to go off. I drift out of sleep with the thoughts of the list of things to do today. Get up and get to my mat before my daughter and son wake up. How long will I get today? One hour? Maybe ten minutes? *Should I skip it...I could do so many other things before I rush off to work.*

The tango of discussion begins in my head: A load of laundry, get the school bags together, enjoy a cup of coffee, check and respond to work emails, or practice yoga. The job I love and have worked so hard to get is also one of the demands that takes me away from my children, my husband, myself, and my time. There are not enough hours in the day. First, my mind thinks and asks, *I have to do it all...can I do it all today? Only the next 24 hours will let me know.* But next, I ask myself a more important question, *does it all have to get done?* This is probably the most important lesson I've learned. No, it doesn't. The alarm rings again.

I rise. Practice has won over tasks. I grab my mat and unroll it. The sound of it hitting the ground is a sound that I've grown to look forward to. It's my time right now—my practice and two fur-ball feline distractions. They know the routine and like to play the game. They seem to say, *I will sit here on your mat and I will get pushed away but it won't stop me from trying.*

I sit and close my eyes to set my intention. A cat rubs his face against my hand as he sets his intention also. New questions arise in my mind, *What will this practice bring? Will I be able to clear my thoughts and focus on my breath?* I begin to breathe, building my internal fire as I prepare to move.

I've been practicing for about fifteen years now and took teacher training in New York City in 2007. I can sequence and I feel that was one of my strong suits during my training. Sequencing is picking a peak pose and building toward it. During a sequence, I can push myself to the breaking point and then calm myself back to a controlled breath. My sun salutes become long and complex. I sweat and pause...a thought of work sneaks into my practice. I start to move again to get back to the task at hand. I move with my breath in a yoga dance that's probably not as graceful as I imagine but it's my practice. This is my moment, and I don't take for granted any movement my body allows. I appreciate my body and thank it each day with my morning practice.

I jump through and come to seated postures preparing to twist and bind. Happiness runs over me and I smile. *Is it because my practice is coming to an end? Perhaps I've physically worked myself into a bit of mental clearness? Maybe the joy is that I adore twists and folds or because I can sit down.* Probably, its source is a bit of them all. With each breath, I remind myself to inhale and extend through my spine, and then to exhale and twist deeper. For me, twists and folds are deeply rewarding. The progress is felt and seen each time I breathe. Maybe that's why I am smiling.

I lie down in final resting savasana and the thoughts creep back in: *Get the kids up, dressed, make breakfast, get the husband up, school run, commute, work, deadline for pitch looming, did I put into the calendar our weekend plans, add dish soap to grocery order, must buy socks for Elle. Stop!* I tell myself to stop and clear my mind again for five minutes.

My mind settles...total clarity. Nothing but clear calm, quiet, and my breath. Success. This is the moment I dream of and why I practice. It's not to get into that wicked asana I saw or to become a super yogi—my practice is to clear the chaos and just be with myself.

Every morning it's a similar sequence of events. As long as I get to my mat for any length of time, I feel my intention has been set. I am just as important as everyone else in my family. I deserve time for me, and my practice allows me to spoil myself a little. I realize that *I'm thinking this* so my mind's clearness has faded but the good vibes remain.

I hear a door open and little feet run toward me. I'm ready. Let's rock this day.

Untitled
Poetry by Lily Gomez

1.
Fold to serve.
Not to submit.
To strengthen.
Not to silence.
To suspend.
Not to surrender.

2.
It is all within reach
If you
Step aside and just
Believe.

3.
I found myself trying to hold water in my hands.
When I arrived, I had nothing.
But as I looked back, everything had drunk
From the droplets I had carried.
When I arrived, I had everything.

4.
Never aspire to be someone else.
Your dharma was uniquely ingrained into your
Breath... And that belongs only to you.
So live to be you.
Dream to be you.
Breathe to be
You.

A Kiss
Nonfiction by Selwa Mitchell

Lying in my own darkness, I listen to his breath. I try to match the rhythm of my breath to his. His deep-sounding breath is so alive and real. I could almost name each breath as they slowly slip out of his mouth. Each one is born from his lungs. Every breath fills his body with serenity, leaving its mark of fulfillment and then saying goodbye with a kiss. Cleansing his soul as it disappears forever.

How I wish my breath would kiss *my* lips. Every breath from my lungs is a humbling reminder that I am not well. As I work for my breath, that humbling reminder turns into and sets off an alarm of panic. Familiar with the panic, I begin calming my mind with words that must come from deep within my soul.

"You are breathing. Air is coming in. You are alive." These words feel like lies, but I continue the lies until my mind takes them as truth. The words slowly create calm while my breath gives none. Every breath I have taken since infancy has been a fight but an understood blessing. At the age of three, I watched my parents' world crumble in a cold, hospital room as doctors told them my diagnosis that I had a rare genetic disorder called cystic fibrosis (CF).

Cystic fibrosis is a progressive genetic disorder that attacks the lungs, slowly and painfully, as well as the pancreas, liver, kidneys, and more and more of the body. There is no cure. CF patients eventually seek lung transplants hoping to add years but knowing that there is no guarantee promised to us. The only guarantee CF patients have is that we are going to die, and quickly, if we don't fight.

As my mind finally quiets, I wipe a tear into my pillow and begin to accept my weak, shallow breath. This is the time to face the inevitability of suffering...time to rise using a broken vessel. For so long, I resented my sick body. I didn't choose this body. It was given to me, and I wanted to give it back.

Until my 200-hour registered yoga training (RYT) two years ago, I considered my body to be the enemy. I understand now that my body was fighting the enemy. Drawing her sword, my body ran straight toward a blood bath of defeat. My body fights with every breath to save my life. The scars my body so proudly wears are scars she took for my life. Despite my cries of despair, my body continues to pump my worn heart, pushing strength into my veins, keeping me alive with every heartbeat. The unconditional love my body gives to me with every beat and breath is a blessing...a gift not to be taken for granted.

To give that love back, I gather all of my strength, mentally and physically, and quietly make my way to my walk-in-closet, trying not to wake my husband. Gasping for air, I quickly inhale the solution from my nebulizer and then attach myself to my vest, putting in the connecting tubes to the machine.

As the lung treatment begins to clear my airways, I cough hard and strong. I giggle at myself as I mentally compliment my "six-pack abs." I refer to them as my "coughing abs." So many people give sanction to my fit body. Women would compliment my beauty and obsess over my thin frame, not realizing this physically comes with a price. They didn't realize it was like a demon starving me from the inside. This disease attacks my digestive system as well as my lungs, making it impossible to gain weight. My tiny frame gives no protection. If my disease decides to fight harder, my body would not have any reserves to help me through the battle. My body needs weight but my body uses every calorie to fight this disease—a disease that wants to destroy every part of me.

Cystic fibrosis wants death—never stopping, never giving up. Its goal in life is to destroy me. But I do not destroy easily, and instead I look him right in the eye, give him a side grin, and take a step forward. The hit from CF comes hard. It always does. With every blow, I do the same—smile and step forward. Every punch only strengthens my fight. The disease has brought me to my knees time and time again but only to pray for strength, to stand again, and continue my fight. I know how to fight through the pain and mental anguish this disease causes. I have fought every day for every breath. Even when that breath reminds me that I am slowly suffocating, I still fight for it because no matter how hard, it is still a blessing to breathe and be alive. This is a suffocating blessing—a contradiction that can mess with my mind.

This blessing hurts and plays mind games with my soul, and slowly exhausts my will to live. I've gained measureless strength in the process of accepting this contradiction—proving that the mind is a powerful tool. My mind knows how to play the game now, and so I tell anyone who ever feels sorry for me, "Don't!"

My struggle has shaped me into my true self. A journey of struggle teaches appreciation, and there is power in that knowledge. I wake up appreciating my very breath, something so simple yet so significant. I wake up with an attitude of gratitude. I am alive! Nothing is going to keep me from happiness because happiness is a choice, and I always choose happiness. If I didn't make this choice, I would die.

Finally finished with my lung treatment, I assess my breathing and fight the discouragement my breath brings. My lungs are still tight and heavy. My body just fought a battle and lost. I want to crawl back in bed, but depression will suck my life away and find ways to suffocate my soul. Instead, I brush my teeth and sigh as I pass my bed. I head into the beautiful kitchen my sweet husband built for me.

Husband, oh sweet husband—a title he so rightfully earned. He is a husband so healthy and strong with a sweet smile and quiet disposition. He doesn't say much, but when he does, I listen, learn, and love. The man has been to more doctor appointments since he married me than for himself in his lifetime. He has busted through those emergency room doors, carrying me so close to his chest that I could feel his frantic heartbeat as he desperately begged someone to fix his wife. The man would die for me and then come back from the grave and do it all over again. I grin at the thought of the face he would make right now if he knew I was popping pain meds and skipping breakfast to make sure I got in my quiet yoga time before our sweet miracle babies wake up with their demands.

Still in yoga pants and tank from the previous day, I quietly place my mat on the dark hardwood floors in the open foyer of my house, feeling the wind from my mat tickle my toes. My insides start to smile. Gently with intention, I lay my body on my mat in my favorite pose—wide child's pose—a rejuvenating, calming pose that allows me to breathe into my torso and relax my lungs. Immediately my body sinks into the mat, my mind quiets, and my soul awakens. Moving on the mat has always come naturally to me.

I attribute my easy transition into yoga to my dance background. Being a child with CF, it was extremely important to stay active and use my lungs to the fullest to keep them strong. My scared and loving parents threw me into everything to keep me active and alive. I smile at the thought of my family. I'm a fighter but this fight cannot be fought alone. With no apparent energy left to stand, my childhood friends would give the effort of their feet. With a stained soul, I could take their last tears. Always fighting alongside me, the asking was challenging at first, but I learned that it's necessary to survive. Doing life alone will not work.

Now in downward-facing dog, I enjoy the weight off my chest and the feel of lengthening my spine. This pose saved me many times while teaching yoga classes. I would become too breathless to speak during my class. Downdog would take the weight off of my chest, open up my airways, and allow me to breathe in a deeper inhale, giving me a chance to catch my breath. Then, I could finish teaching and do what I was born to do—share the love of yoga.

I thank God every day for giving me the gift of yoga. Yoga has taught me so much about who I am and what I need. It creates a desire in me to find my full potential. Yoga awakens the beast inside. Every day I wake and wonder what secret jewels I will find hidden so deep inside. This is a thought that drives me to greatness. With every pose, with every breath, the jewels begin to rise up out of the darkness and fuel the light that reveals my potential. Every challenge and every test introduces me to my true body...my true self beyond.

Certainly, we know our bodies can walk, run, or pick up heavy things. The questions are how long can we walk, how fast can we run, or how heavy can we lift. Those challenges and tests drive us to meet goals. Those goals push us to work hard and the working hard builds our true character, creates health, and opens the door to our soul; thus, creating wellness.

That morning in the foyer on my mat, I decide to seek my handstand press. This is a flow that requires every part of my body, mind, and soul to be in sync and united. I slowly bend over and press my palms to the earth and begin to press my body up into the air. Stacking my shoulders over my wrists, my hips over my shoulders, like magic, I float. My legs feel weightless as they flow up to the sky. My body creates a straight line upside-down. Defying gravity, peace flows through my veins. My blood rushes through my body. With every muscle engaged, the noise stops. I practice this handstand flow over and over again until I cannot get it wrong. An hour of bliss seeps into my soul, forever embedded into my heart, and offering strength for my fight with a disease.

Resting on my mat with a sheen of sweat covering my skin, I relish the bliss that my quiet mind left behind. The diseased girl is gone and replaced with a woman who can hold herself up, defy gravity and disease, and float with my breath again and again. I smile. Lying in my inner light, I listen to my breath kiss my lips.

Sitting in the Mud
Nonfiction by Leslie Storms

Yoga has lovingly taught me the importance of learning to sit with discomfort. I am reminded of the lotus flower that births itself from within the mud. No one escapes the reality that life is sometimes uncomfortable and painful.

When that pain/discomfort arrives, we all have certain patterns of responding. These predictable patterns are rooted in the ego and are most often subliminally learned from society. As soon as we notice a hint of discomfort, we unconsciously launch into fleeing from the pain. We attempt to fix, control, blame, deny, and even withdraw. Our egos will go to great extremes to avoid experiencing pain.

Yoga has shown me a sacred, transformational space that lives within each of us. This space revealed itself through the daily practice of controlling the breath while placing the body in uncomfortable poses. Putting the body in awkward poses creates the ideal conditions to trigger the ego. Suddenly the ego is screaming, "~let me out~!"

Yet, if a yoga practitioner remains patient and focused, the breath will softly override the ego's demand to be freed. It is an indescribable space where the body connects to a vastness. I refer to it as Spirit or God.

How does this apply off the mat? When I began to sit with discomforts versus making an attempt to control or dissolve them, ~ a similar space began to open.

For example, if you experience pain and you begin to resist that pain, you are simply adding to your suffering, because now you have pain as well as a desire to be free from the pain. Whereas, if you silently think, *I am feeling pain. Can I go straight into the pain and allow it to be there without all the negative mind chatter like judgments, evaluations, and questions that want it to go away?*, and if you sincerely commit to this path—the Truth will begin to reveal itself. The Truth is that you hold the key to end your suffering. The Truth is that transformations take place in our most painful occurrences. The Truth is that our most natural state is free from the ego's demands and that an infinite love is just a breath away.

Instead of responding through a desperate desire to be free from pain, anxieties, fears, and doubts, you learn to pour yourself deeply into the muck. And, while metaphorically covered in mud, you can begin to really allow the reality of what you are experiencing. You can then silently ask yourself: *What is behind this experience?*

There is a phrase: Each emotion we experience has come here to teach us something. I would add: If we are brave enough to sit in the midst of discomfort.

All Because She Tried
Poetry by Jacquitta Boone

She Fell.
After finally learning how to enter this pose properly,
And finally learning how to breathe in it,
She Fell.
Perplexed at how, even with all the right tools, she could still fail,
She lay there, with a feeling of defeat.
How could she not nail this pose?
The same pose that everyone around her seemed to get.
The same pose that she nailed before but suddenly could
Not
Nail
Again....

She continued to lie there,
Contemplating whether she should try again.
The fall was not her focus,
However,
Rebuilding her confidence was.
Suddenly a still small voice told her to
"Try Again."
Still unsure, she couldn't help but think about falling again and hurting
Herself
Again
But the still small voice interrupted and whispered,
"Try again."
So she meditated,
Regained her composure,
And tried again....

This time with a newfound confidence,
Not knowing that she could do it,
But knowing that she could not give up,
No matter who told her she couldn't,
No matter what made her think she couldn't,

And no matter how many times she failed.
She picked herself up,
Took a deep breath,
And as she exhaled all of her frustrations,
She tried again...

This time
Working her way into the pose,
While taking deep breaths
And focusing her energy in all the right places—

She
Nailed
It.

Without even noticing, she held this position for a couple of breaths.
Afterwards, feeling invigorated,
She slowly worked her way out of the pose and smiled from the depths
Of her soul.
She had a new confidence,
Knowing that she could do anything,
Absolutely anything, if she just took the first step.
It was all because she tried.

Yoga Fills My Hole
Nonfiction by Katie Schroeder

I have a permanent hole in my abdomen…that poop comes out of—yes, I said it, poop, crap, shit, waste, feces, whatever you want to call it. And yoga helped me survive until I finally got the "poop hole" that saved my life. Yoga made me realize that I wouldn't live to see twenty-nine years old unless I got my permanent ileostomy (the "poop hole"), even if having life-changing and body-altering surgeries meant risking never being able to return to the intense asana practice I had developed since first toying with yoga in my early teens. Without my yoga practice, I wouldn't be alive today, I wouldn't have gained the body awareness that shocks doctors, I wouldn't have learned to appreciate rather than hate the chronic illnesses I've had my entire life and developed later on, I wouldn't hang on when others might give up, I wouldn't have found my passion and mission in life, I wouldn't have found myself, and I wouldn't have my ostomy, which I named Marvin.

Always the shy girl with the tummy ache who spent hours in the bathroom, embarrassed to go on sleepovers or miss an entire class because of my chronic constipation, I grew up feeling like I was always hiding a secret that no one would understand. My family knew if I had to have a bowel movement, it would be a thirty-minute or longer ordeal, which made me feel guilty on road trips or other outings. That guilt is still with me today. Rumors spread in grade school, high school, and around the area where I grew up, that I was anorexic or bulimic because eating meant having to spend up to an hour in the bathroom, and I dropped almost thirty pounds in a short period of time.

I've always been a health nut and tried to eat a very healthy diet. But eating hurt, and I couldn't explain to people why I rarely ate lunch in high school or why I always turned down going out to restaurants with the supposed girlfriends who ultimately abandoned me, choosing to believe what they saw instead of learning who I was inside. I was socially isolated, bullied, and suffering in silence. Relatives, those who are supposed to love and support you, judged me, made snide comments, and left me behind too.

I had my first colonoscopy, a procedure most don't have until their forties or fifties, at the age of fifteen. I've had three colonoscopies and several other gruesome, painful medical tests multiple times at several hospitals in which doctors poke and prod at places people are afraid to talk about and that required prep methods that still nauseate me just thinking about them. After my first colonoscopy, when I had a massive fecal impaction (hardened stool clogged up in my digestive tract), I was told that I had constipation-prone Irritable Bowel Syndrome and to increase my fiber intake. That was a disaster, yet I still couldn't get my head to listen to my body and realize that raw produce and high fiber foods were making things worse.

It was then that I started meditating every night, gazing at a candle, as calming techniques were supposed to help my digestive tract get going. I stayed active, running in cross-country and track, excelling in school, taking leading roles in several clubs, working two jobs, and had to plan all these activities around my bowel movements. To this day, doctors and I don't know how I survived all of that given what was going on with my body.

The best thing I ever did in high school was buying my first yoga book and that started a nightly routine that I stuck to religiously. It became my anchor, shutting myself in my room late at night, breathing, moving, stretching, and meditating. I would forget how alone I felt, how much I wished I could have a "normal" teenage life filled with dating and late nights instead of having to get up at five a.m. every day to make sure I had enough time to empty my gut as much as possible before enduring a long day (usually with no food) until I'd be alone and have time to spend hours pushing and straining on the toilet. I did my homework in the bathroom. Most don't know that's how this valedictorian studied. Still, that nightly routine of yoga, as simple as it was then, was my rock and filled the holes in my life.

The first truly, freeing, happy time of my life was my freshman year of college, when I escaped my hometown, left all those rumors and started fresh. I was on a medication that helped me get through my first year, I made friends and became known as "the girl from the gym" or the "yoga girl" practicing in dorm common areas. All of that changed at the beginning of my sophomore year. If I wasn't in class, at the gym, tutoring athletes, or practicing my vinyasas in the dorm, I was in the bathroom. I pushed people away, never went out, and spent my weekends at the local bookstore studying. I lost friends and all wondered what happened to the girl who loved to dance all night, then hop on the treadmill just hours later, the *"Oh my God, Hi!"* girl who was always smiling.

My weight was dropping drastically again. The isolation returned, but yoga filled that void. If I didn't do my daily practice, I didn't feel calm and whole. My stomach began to hurt more and more, I couldn't eat more than a bite of food without feeling full and enduring severe pain. I planned on switching majors, leaving behind my dreams of entering the medical field because I couldn't handle the long science labs with my digestive system. But then I ended up withdrawing from the school that I loved and still miss, where I could have built a new life as my parents said when they dropped me off my freshman year: "She's never coming back. She's going to get married out there, become an amazing doctor, and finally be happy."

I traveled home during fall break to have an emergency colonoscopy that left the gastroenterologist perplexed. After returning to school and receiving the phone call from the doctor that turned my world upside down, I felt lost and broken. I couldn't continue living the way I was, in the bathroom five or more hours a day. I made the hardest decision of my life—harder than deciding to get my ostomy—and decided to withdraw from college. When my mom flew out to help me move home, she said that I looked like a ghost, pale and frail, weak with no spark left.

Yoga continued to be the one thing keeping me going while I went through several tests to finally get a diagnosis of Hypertonic Pelvic Floor Dysfunction. The muscles in my pelvic floor never worked correctly since my first bowel movement as an infant because I was born with a very crooked pelvis. I never knew the pain all over my body was chronic muscle tension instead of general soreness from daily runs and gym workouts until a physical therapist first examined me and started attempting to massage the knots in my pelvis (yes, inside too...pelvic floor physical therapy isn't pretty), butt, thighs, abdomen, and lower back. I was diagnosed with gastroparesis—stomach paralysis—and osteoporosis at the young age of nineteen after suffering my first of about seven stress fractures from running and an acroyoga/cheerleading stunt.

Over the next ten years, top physical therapists gave up on me because my muscles wouldn't relax enough to let stool and urine pass easily, and intense medications and prescribed laxatives left me depressed and bed-ridden for six months. I tried to work and return to school while juggling physical therapy and doctors' appointments, maintaining an active lifestyle, but still ended up having to withdraw from school twice more before finally finishing my degree. I couldn't manage to hold down a job for more than a few months. My interest in yoga grew stronger when I backed away from modern medicine because they refused to repair my permanently damaged right hip when I cracked my pelvis on its weakest side. I said, "Enough's enough. I can't take another doctor jumping to conclusions about me, accusing me of having an eating disorder; and I can't take being let down yet again."

Studying yoga instead of general fitness started to make things click for me. Discovering Ayurveda—yoga's sister science—helped me to see what conventional medicine was missing and helped me understand my illness more as I found out that I have an extremely strong *vata dosha*. Vata is one of the three Ayurvedic principles in the body, and vata leads the mind and body by controlling waste eliminations, blood flow, breathing, and thought patterns.

Thankfully, I was able to focus on yoga for women's health as my final college project. Whatever paper or project I was assigned, I made it about yoga as my daily practice grew stronger and I began taking regular ashtanga classes. I was able to see the connections between all of the muscles that physical therapists focused on during our sessions and why many of the exercises they prescribed were basically asanas.

Yoga confirmed my belief that the body is a whole connected entity, not separate parts as Western medicine treats it. Instead of torturing myself at the gym, I gave up running and lifting, and focused solely on yoga and walking. Even a permanent shoulder injury didn't stop me from studying and practicing as I learned modifications and proper alignment during my yoga teacher training. While some yoga teachers would try to force one side of my body to exactly match the other, my teacher trainer helped me not only to modify my practice to suit my unique crooked body but also to appreciate and even laugh at the differences between sides.

Going through my teacher training was truly life-changing, even though I had to do it yet again on little food and while maintaining a full time job in a busy city. My home practice grew stronger on my mat. More importantly, my outlook on life shifted. I was able to see my health struggles as blessings in disguise as I studied the *Yoga Sutra* and other yoga books, the chakras, and Ayurveda. I was able to achieve a sense of calm in the midst of chaos, pause before reacting and reach a deep level of gratitude for the small things in life that most take for granted and for the multiple ways my immediate family supported me—with everything from picking me up off the floor when intense medications made me pass out several times in the middle of the night, to helping me financially when I couldn't work enough to pay for school and make a living. I was happy, spreading smiles, and socializing again. Yoga was filling the cracks in my life.

Then, life changed again. Looking back, I know it was because I was caught on the wrong path, working a high-stress office job that prevented me from seeking my true passion of teaching yoga and spreading awareness of Pelvic Floor Dysfunction and how yoga can help treat it. I once again ended up searching for help from highly-esteemed doctors, had multiple tests done, was hospitalized, and came so close to getting the surgery I had been begging for since I was fifteen—an ileostomy. I hit a brick wall with yet another doctor who didn't understand that I had been suffering for well over twenty years, that things were getting worse daily, and that I couldn't live on laxatives and enemas indefinitely.

Even though my quality of life was non-existent, I still got on my mat daily, even when nauseated from harsh medications and having to take multiple breaks to go to the bathroom. No matter how I felt, if I could flow and get upside down, I knew things were somehow going to be okay, and I felt there must be a reason why I was still living.

When one of the top surgeons in the area neglected to see the severity of my condition, I went through intense self-treatment using Ayurveda, yoga, pranayama, and meditation. I researched and tried several healing diets—everything from The Gut and Psychology Syndrome Diet (GAPS), The Specific Carbohydrate Diet (SCD), vegan, to Paleolithic and Paleo vegan. My body and mind started going crazy, my hormones were out of whack, and I hadn't had a regular period since my early teens. I kept losing weight and still had to take megadoses of laxatives every week and do Ayurvedic and conventional enemas almost daily just so that I could leave my apartment. Being jolted awake daily at 3:00 a.m. feeling like someone was kicking and stabbing me in the vagina, the place where life is supposed to be given, not taken, was horrific.

I was offended when people stared at me or commented on how they wished they were as "thin" as me. In my head, I was thinking *I wish I could eat and have a pain-free, fucking bowel movement like you.* Prejudgments like that are one of the few things that make me angry because of all I've been through to find answers. I had no social life, couldn't work, but I had yoga to fulfill me. Meditating longer each day helped me with the physical and emotional pain. However, I needed a change as the cold weather in the Midwest made my chronic muscle tension and digestive problems worse.

I moved to the Southeast, which was a second home to me, and the humid, salty, ocean air was a warm hug that relaxed my muscles. I hoped for a new future, teaching yoga, writing, and building true relationships. Yet again, my body was still in turmoil. I couldn't eat without having to give myself enemas (I was a pro), my herbal remedies and supplements weren't working anymore, I had to take laxatives daily, and the pelvic pain worsened. I called my mom, my best friend who always fights for me when I can't stand up for myself to doctors, and we knew this was it...I wasn't going to live another six months unless they gave me an ostomy and removed my colon that was wreaking havoc on my body, causing years of malnutrition due to its inability to function properly.

I clung to my yoga practice like a child holds her teddy bear, practicing as much as I could because I was afraid I'd lose my asana practice. I worried that having an ileostomy and wearing a "bag" (ostomy pouch/appliance) would mean *sayonara* to backbends, prone postures, twists, arm balances, and inversions. On my last beach walk before flying to my hometown to see my main gastroenterologist, I saw my beloved dolphins. Knowing they magically appeared to tell me I was making the right decision, I burst into tears.

Thankfully, my gastroenterologist understood that I was at wit's end and referred me to the newly-appointed Chief of Colorectal Surgery at the main hospital where I had been treated—a brilliant kind man who is one of the best colorectal surgeons in the country. His first words to me after reading my novel of a health history were: "I get it." It was a huge relief to finally find a doctor who understood why I needed this operation. He was able to squeeze me in a couple weeks later.

I practiced yoga as much as possible and had a marathon photo session with my mom. She surprised me with a collage video of all my yoga pictures that I could watch and remember the feeling of my beloved practice in case I could never do those postures again. Immediately after my first surgery, I woke up groggy and knew right away that my pelvis was finally happy.

I had several complications post-op that my yoga-induced body intuition helped me to convince doctors that something was wrong. I tried relieving ostomy blockages and gas and mucus built up in my colon, that was still inside me, with simple postures such as *virasana* (hero pose) with deep breathing. I even managed to get into *viparita karani* (legs-up-the-wall pose) less than 24-hours after surgery while all hooked up to an IV and catheter in order to try to relieve the pressure in my colon. My doctors and nurses were baffled that I was elated to have my ostomy that I eventually named Marvin, after Marvin the Martian because I described him as an alien poking out of me! I eventually had a second surgery in which my surgeon removed my colon and rectum and sealed everything up down there, giving me what ostomates jokingly call a "Barbie Butt."

All in all, I had two major surgeries, six emergency room visits (one by ambulance at 2:00 a.m.), six hospital stays, bed rest for six weeks, and a five-month break from my yoga practice. And yet, I was able to eat comfortably for the first time in my life. It took weeks to get my weight into the triple digits. During my bed-ridden weeks, I read books about yoga, and although it saddened me because I worried that I'd never be able to get out of bed and actually function, seeing other yogis practice left a spark of hope. That spark ignited into a bright fire when my surgeon gave me the okay to gradually resume my practice.

As much of a struggle as it was, I've always appreciated the times I had to treat myself as a beginner again. I always learn something new, especially when I had to learn how to modify poses and what to wear when practicing yoga with an ostomy. I remember crying when attempting *chaturanga dandasana* (four-limbed staff pose, also known as low plank pose) again after surgery because I'd lost all strength in my arms and core and had to practice with my knees down for weeks until the risk of hurting Marvin and getting a hernia decreased. Those tears turned into happy ones when I inverted for the first time after my surgeries in *sirsana* (tripod headstand).

The struggle with backbends was the most challenging, as even *setu bandha sarvangasana* (supported bridge pose) worried me that I'd stretch Marvin too much or risk my ostomy bag coming off. It was incredibly difficult for the hard-headed type A person that I am to be patient and not push myself too much, too soon. Slowly, as my practice became stronger again, I returned to life in a new way, with a new body and stoma buddy, Marvin. Yoga was filling not just emotional holes but my new physical "poop hole."

After moving back to the South in the summer of 2014, I discovered Instagram and found a huge, online yoga community in these little photo squares. I started joining a few challenges to help me continue to get my practice back. At the same time, I applied for and landed what I thought was my dream job, and I started socializing. The friendships I made through the Instagram yoga community have been life-changing and life-saving. Those yogis, near and far, helped me get over my fears of falling and helped me break up with "Paul the Wall." Moving my handstand practice away from the wall gave me a reputation for my ability to hold handstands for a long time.

The Instagram community stuck with me even when I couldn't stay in touch as my job took up most of my time. Yet, I continued to practice daily and join challenges when possible. I made a pact with myself to never give up, once I got my little Marvin. I never dropped out of a yoga challenge, even if I wasn't feeling well. I only took breaks from my first year of handstands when my job landed me in the hospital twice due to severe dehydration, exhaustion, and inability to eat.

A true blessing entered my life when I connected with the inspiring woman who became my stoma sister after someone referred her to my Instagram page. She had just found out that she needed a permanent ostomy and was worried that she'd lose her physical practice, too. I was able to show her that all of the asanas that I was afraid I would have to give up were still possible, and that my practice actually grew stronger because I was healthier and not living on medications and laxatives anymore. We helped each other during her ostomy surgery and each of our recurring hospital stays. We hope to inspire other ostomates that practicing yoga, and living and thriving with an ostomy are not out of reach. Without her kindness and support and without the connections with sincere yogis from all over the world, I wouldn't have gathered the courage to leave the job that was killing me and pursue my true passions of writing, teaching yoga, and helping other ostomates realize that life doesn't end when getting that "poop hole" but often begins in a new magical way.

There have been times when I've doubted my purpose in this world: when I struggle with my ostomy because I eat the wrong foods, don't hydrate enough, or feel down due to giving up hope for a romantic relationship because I don't want to force a guy to deal with Marvin. Yet, every morning when I step on my mat, I'm reminded that I should be grateful to be alive and to be able to practice yoga, for my ability to maintain a consistent daily practice, as I know there are many who can't and wish they could. I've been *there*, stuck in bed with hard wiry stitches poking out of my sealed-up "Barbie Butt," having endured crawling from my bedroom to the bathroom because I couldn't stand upright, due to nauseating medications. My diagnosis and treatment were long overdue, so there is damage to my body that will never be undone. Eating is still a struggle, my bones are still weak, my hormones are irregular, but I'm alive.

I always remind myself of what my teacher during yoga training taught me: *If you can breathe, you can do yoga.* It's not about the fancy poses, how strong or "flexi" the pose is, or how your body looks, it's about how you *feel*. I'm grateful to feel alive every day when I breathe and move, and Marvin loves yoga! He loves when I take deep calming breaths, as I still have chronic muscle tension that can choke him. He loves when I turn my body upside down and gets "excited"—this is my way of saying that he "goes" (empties poop into his "home", my ostomy bag), for which I'm always grateful because the sluggishness in my stomach and small intestine is something I'll have to deal with forever.

Despite fearing that backbends would be impossible with an ostomy, my heart-opening practice has deepened immensely. I couldn't have progressed with Marvin in my yoga practice without the inspiration and motivation I've been given by the wonderful yogis I've met all over the world. Yoga is filling the emptiness that I felt in unexpected ways.

Again, it's not about the poses—it is about how yoga makes me feel. Yoga is about feeling whole, at home in my body, with its "poop hole" and all its crookedness. It is about laughing when I fall out of an inversion, and it's about connecting with myself and others. It's about doing what makes me feel full. It's about feeling like I was given the body I have for a specific reason. That reason comes to life and warms my heart when ostomates reach out to me with questions, and when nurses show new ostomates my pictures to encourage them.

Yoga has filled the gaping holes in my life since the day I picked up my first yoga book and now fills the lingering emotional holes, the physical hole that is now a permanent part of my life, and the sometimes empty feelings that come with it. Yoga kept me alive until Marvin saved me, continues to keep me thriving, led me to my purpose, and helps me love living with an ostomy.

BE
Poetry by Jasmin Serina

Mind and body

Peaceful beauty

You are thinking

You are moving

Breathing... breathing

Meditating

Forever be

The Bridge
Nonfiction by Deb Harano

Many years ago as a young woman, I was vaguely aware of this deep longing to practice yoga. At the time, I truly did not understand what that meant, only that I had a desire which lay in wait. Many years would pass before I actually came to my mat for the first time. Finally, in middle age, after the births of children, the drama of divorce, stress of relocation, fear of re-marriage and a variety of careers, I finally stood on my mat for the very first time. I noticed a sense of anticipation, but also a sense of peace as I stood in the cool basement, feet placed carefully in the first of many mountain poses. I believe in perfect timing, and while part of me knew this moment would come eventually, I had no idea what standing on that mat on that particular morning would inspire.

Often I am asked how long I've practiced yoga, but I do not know the exact date, month, or year when I first stood there. Perhaps I would have paid closer attention had I known that it would be a life-changing event. I came to my mat one quiet morning at home, with a carefully chosen DVD to practice ashtanga with Nicki Doane. She would be my first teacher. I chose this particular style for its "vigorous" practice and if I'm honest, I also wanted to make sure I would get a good "workout," as I love a challenge. The idea of consistency was also attractive. I took comfort in knowing what my practice would look like each day and I could practice at home, since there was not a studio nearby where I could practice ashtanga. I listened closely and followed everything, and I mean *everything* Nicki said to do; every breath and each verbal cue was followed as precisely as I was able. Eventually, I practiced religiously and was quite amazed at how I felt afterwards.

After running countless miles throughout my adult life, I was quite familiar with the "runner's high," but was not prepared to have a similar experience on the mat, without running one single step. I was so drawn into this feeling without the miles, and I wanted more. Yoga became my moving meditation, which transported me to places of peace and calm, both mentally and physically. Little did I realize it then, but this was the first step toward coming back to me.

I eventually allowed "life" to pull me away from my blossoming young practice, but when I did return a few years later, my soul leapt for joy, and I wondered why I had left it at all. How could I miss this so desperately and not recognize it was missing? Instead of restarting my home practice, my husband and I joined a gym with its own yoga program. My body was somewhat stiffer and my arm strength had slipped away, but this was a great way to reunite with my practice.

The breath and the movement fulfilled me to the very core of my being and I was immediately enamored. I found my long lost peace as my body literally sighed with relief. I practiced almost daily and often stayed for two classes in a row. I quickly regained my strength and flexibility. The instructors were so kind and supportive, showing me the little places where I needed to pay attention, and were always incredibly encouraging. I was introduced to arm balances that were previously unknown to me and found them to be somewhat natural. Eventually, it became normal to be asked to demonstrate for the class. Believing I was a "shy" person, I surprised myself by agreeing to demonstrate in front of strangers. I even felt at ease as I achieved postures that were new to me. The faith of my teachers had awakened a budding sense of confidence that filled me with gratitude.

My growing practice and deepening need took me to a new studio where the eight limbs of yoga were expressly practiced and this further allowed me to continue to explore my practice in a new and deeper way by offering new variations for familiar postures and introducing me to concepts like the *yamas* and *niyamas* (moral, ethical, and societal "rules" for living that are described in Panatanjali's *Yoga Sutra*). I had found my yoga home, my tribe. After my third class in this new space, I decided to continue to deepen my practice and take their 200-hour yoga teacher training.

In the few months leading up to the training, I had the opportunity to experiment with my physical form and to try postures and variations that I had never before tried. I came to realize that there is always someplace else to take a posture, being inspired by those who shared the practice with me at the studio. I was amazed that, "at my age," I could do things that those much younger than I struggled to achieve. In that studio, no one questioned my abilities, and they even encouraged me to explore my capabilities. My understanding of the eight limbs expanded as well. Before asana, there would always be a short "spiritual" talk and a practice of pranayama. I welcomed these teachings that resonated with me. I had found my path, leaving one behind that no longer served me. There were several other key lessons to embrace, as I came to recognize that yoga is a practice, first and foremost. It is called a "practice" for a reason and that practice might look different day to day. I learned that movement without breath is not yoga. Even if there is no apparent movement, the practice *is* the breath. And, it's so important to understand that we all start somewhere, and where we are in the moment is where we need to be.

Through it all and to my absolute delight, I was reunited with the playful little girl I had so long forgotten, and don't remember laughing so much or having so much fun! My soul soared as I had finally allowed myself to reconnect with the joy that was latent, but waiting for rediscovery. Over the years, I had become so serious and couldn't imagine the idea of failure. In this studio, I learned that it was okay to try—and to fall. Everyone falls sometimes. It wasn't important that I fell, but it mattered that I got back up. I learned to laugh and try again. I practiced at the studio almost daily and I couldn't get enough. Each class held a wonderment of what I might achieve that day.

Eventually, my husband joined me at the studio, and his practice also began to expand and strengthen. He was encouraged to take the teacher training and finally agreed to do so, although he had no intention of teaching at all.

We never really know what the future brings, and the teacher training opened a door and led me to understand that yoga was my path, my dharma, which would become my life itself. It reawakened my sleeping meditation practice and helped me to realize that I experience much more peace when I practice meditation on a regular basis. While I had no serious intentions of teaching after the completion of teacher training, it would be my dear teachers who saw in me more than I had ever seen in myself. They often called on me in training, to nudge me past my limited, self-imposed boundaries, by asking me to do things on the spot, like leading meditation or giving a spiritual talk with no more than a couple of minutes' notice. I had spent much of my life in hiding, both from the world and perhaps hiding from myself. Through my yoga practice, I slowly began to recognize that I could no longer hide and be true to the woman whom I was uncovering and discovering. So, I took a breath and moved forward.

To my surprise, the studio where I trained wanted to hire me after I completed the teacher training, and they made this known to me about halfway through the program. Immediately, I was hired and taught my first class two days after completing the training. I have been teaching there since that time. If it were not for the encouragement and urging of my teachers, I would not have pursued this direction. They changed my life, for I did not see myself as a "teacher." In all honesty, those first months of teaching were formidable. As was my pattern, I continued to question myself, wondering if I was really capable, and if I was worthy to be in the role of a teacher.

Teaching has challenged me to examine my own beliefs about who I thought I was and who I wanted to be. I already knew I was a good student. I now also understand we all are both students and teachers; formally or informally. Some say, that if you are a good student, you can be a good teacher. I can only hope that is true for me, as I continue to hope to be that teacher for those who come to my class. The physical practice is only a small part of what I teach in class. Linking movement with breath is yoga, but asana is merely the frame, a decoration for the breath; for the deeper work that yoga offers is truth. One of my teachers would often say in class that the breath was the bridge between body and spirit.

As I continue to walk this yogic path, my story evolves. The emotional healing I began to seek in my early thirties has continued and will continue through my consistent yoga practice. Some days appear to be more unyielding, and I allow myself to be pulled out of my center, but when these occurrences happen, I now know what I need to do to re-center and ground myself.

Through it all, I feel my authentic self blossoming and basking in the light of love. I am always happy to recognize something in my life that I just didn't quite get previously, and thrilled when I am able to peel back another layer of the distracting barriers of fear and confusion. It is my yoga practice that continues to draw me back to myself over and over again. Isn't that what yoga is about? To join with the higher self that knows only peace, understands love, and can claim the joy of declaring, "I am," in truth. When I can stand in the light, I am able to walk the Earth plane with an expanded consciousness—sharing, learning, and being unconditional love. When life around me seems to be anything but peaceful and calm, I can step back, take a breath, and continue to practice yoga.

Then, I make the space to remind myself of these words from the *Yoga Sutra,* YS1.2, *"Yogash chitta vritti nirodaha."*
One translation by Swami Rama is as follows:
"Yoga stills the fluctuations of the mind. Yoga is the mastery of the activities of the mind-field. Then the seer rests in its very true nature."

Truly, my yoga practice led me back to my authentic self. For years, I longed to find relief from the ideas of mass consciousness and societal norms. Much of the journey was helpful, from friends and church, to therapy and self-help books, but it was the yoga that truly reunited me with my higher self.

While my longing for relief may not have been conscious at first, I can see now that was the point of all of it—to come to this place of self-discovery, self-acceptance, and self-love. There is nothing selfish about this. As I arrived to myself, I recognized that this is where it must begin in each moment. The more I have within, the more I can offer to the world. From this place of my higher self, I can reflect to others the truth of who they are. My teachers reflected myself to me, and not as I saw myself, but as they saw me. I was finally ready to consider what they saw and now this is what I see. This role of teacher, as guide and facilitator, is an honor for me. I enjoy only opening the door and guiding, as the student must walk through and discover her truth for herself.

Living Bigger
Poetry by Bonnie Weeks

Being spiritual
Was being religious;
That's what I thought.
But when my religion
Began to have holes,
I wasn't held up.

At first I could reconcile
And just ignore it,
But with so much untruth
I just couldn't sit.
What was being spiritual
If religion wasn't it?

My heart was heavy,
This was all I knew.
How could this
Have been made up?
How could this be untrue?
Does it matter if it is?
Is it possible to be part
Being okay
If you're misunderstood?

The answer was no.
Because I had no peace.
My brain was in turmoil,
Where was the release?
I needed to stop pretending,
It's no way to live.

I found yoga.
Or yoga found me.
It answered my questions
My doubts and my fears.

It reminded me of love and
Letting go
And being right here.

Yoga gave me a fire.
It said, "Move in this space,
See your good,
Spread that,
Sit with your heart,
Live big.
Do you see it?
You are enough.
Now share."

I slowed down,
I released my grip.
It was okay.
I am okay.
I felt peace.

Having all the answers
Isn't important.
Spirituality is lifting
Where you stand,
To keep moving forward,
Mindful of where I am.

I don't know tomorrow
Or the ways that I'll change,
But as I love and
Am loved,
My home remains.

The Current
Nonfiction by Nikki Martin

I wrote a story about a girl named Evan McBride. The most beautiful things about her life were the things that didn't happen to her. It was as if the world, and life, moved around her, and then past her, like she was a large immovable rock in a river...always left behind by those cascading currents in their journey forward, onward, home.

I didn't realize at the time I was writing a story about myself and all the space I'd placed between me and the world, to keep from getting hurt, to avoid feeling too deeply and loving too intimately, and of knowing too much in the only way truly sensitive people can. And so the story I wrote for Evan was much like my life. I placed happiness, adventure, and love, and all of the wonderful things we experience in our lifetime all around Evan, and yet forever just out of reach. And like me, though a little bit sad and lonely, she revelled in her safety and what she thought could be the happy life of an observer. Evan never made it to her thirties. That was not the life that I wrote for her. But I did make it to that decade of my life. And in my thirties, something changed....

I had always been drawn to yoga. There was an unseen magnetism that had me orbiting the whole of it for years; I'd been a moon waltzing around and around it, forever drawn but still distant, with no desire to escape its pull. In 2012, I finally surrendered to that gravity and unknowingly stepped onto another path—one that would let me touch the world, one that would finally carry me downstream.

I began my yoga practice that fall with a fervor I had rarely known. I watched a video a few weeks prior called *The Aerialist* in which a woman yogi moved through a ballet-like sequence of arm balances, inversions, and other poses. I don't know why but something inside me broke at the beauty and elegance of it and then somehow it all fell back together again in a new and different way, so that I was whole and yet changed. I decided, even though I'd never been that fit or graceful, that I would try to do what she could, no matter how long it took. So, three times a week, I went to yoga with the desire to learn and know and experience it all burning inside me. I was spurred on by the progress of my body and the slow but steady changes in my mind, heart, and soul.

I began to understand something I hadn't. That the fear of every damn thing I'd had up until then—the fear of failing or falling, of being hurt, of feeling foolish, of discomfort and even pain, of loving and being loved—well, that fear wasn't protecting me at all, and it had kept me locked away and had prevented me from living any kind of life that I could look back on and admire or even celebrate.

My yoga practice increased. Four times a week, then five, six, and yet the stronger and surer and more capable I became, the less I needed to be that woman in the video, and the more I simply needed to discover the very best version of myself.

That beginning was almost four years ago. I'm not sure there are enough words or time for me to really tell you all that I have gotten and learned to give through this life-altering practice of yoga. Yet, I know this...yoga has been a practice in remembering and forgetting, and then remembering again. The yoga practice is a kind of unraveling of all the layers and lies that I had wrapped around myself to stay safe and to be strong. Yoga has been a drawing back beyond all the pain, torment, and terror of the past to the person who can love and live without fear, to the person who I was when I first stepped into this lifetime of mine.

Yoga has torn me down in the most humbling of ways, and then built me back up through my own passion, persistence, and determination. My yoga practice has taught me to let go and how to move on. My practice allowed me to know, for sure, that I am whole with or without my achievements and accomplishments. Yoga has given the knowledge that I am enough, just as I am, even as I strive to be better. It has allowed me to tear down the walls around my heart and embrace my ability to feel so very deeply. I love fully as every heart and soul is destined, with abandon and grace, so that now I am as I was always meant to be, as we all are. I am not a rock in a stream with no hope of moving forward, instead I am the very stream itself, part of that current of life and light, hurrying onward, winding its way home.

The Return to Self
Poetry by Jessica Ruby Hernandez

Self bleeds into my mind's eye.
I lick my lips, enjoying the taste
Of freedom
As I let go of control.
Giving my mind, presenting it
In a purple box
To the bigger Me
As a gift,
A sacrifice,
To appease the Soul
That waits
With open arms
And open heart
For my much anticipated return.
I dwell here forevermore.

Being the Mountain
Nonfiction by Lois McAffrey-Lopez

I often begin my yoga practice with *tadasana*, mountain pose, which is a place of strength, equanimity, and stability.

Coming into the pose, I turn my focus first to my inward self, as I stand tall with arms loose at my side. My breath is relaxed and even. I feel the ground, sure beneath my feet. I begin to feel energy, like my breath, coursing through my body. I feel solid. A knowing begins. Knowing I belong in this moment, in this place. There is space for me, and I hold awareness of it with a joy beyond words. I must simply BE.

There is a natural curve in my back, and I feel it lengthen as I breathe deeply into the space. I feel my head and neck relax, balanced lightly over my body. I feel the breath equally in the front and back, from side to side, making space within my body and allowing me to claim my rightful home, here, on this earth.

Once, in my first year of yoga, as I struggled through a beginner's workshop in my normal, clenched-fist manner, the instructor walked softly behind me and touched my back lightly as I struggled to perform. "Breathe. Feel your back ribs expand," and for a startled moment I thought, "*Back* ribs?"

For so much of my life, I had been living in the abstract experience of my thoughts, disconnected from a sense of my body as a space I might inhabit. I observed my body and I cared for my body, but I lived in a body without interior space, as flat, as lifeless, as the images on a screen.

I find great strength in this inner space, front ribs and back ribs and an infinite world in between. It is here, in this inner world, where strength resides. In my past, I had often confused strength with so-called will power. I believed clenched fists and jaws helped me to give my best efforts, but this was not building strength, only tension.

Strength is to be found in the quiet place of balance, between knowing effort and letting go, between movement and resistance. It cannot be forced and tightly held. In tadasana, I am strong, simply feeling the earth beneath my feet, the strength and length of my body, and my head rising up, light, to the sky. Like a mountain.

The Eyes Do Yoga
Poetry by C.T. Kern

And then there are your eyes.
They should, I suppose, be closed
or focused on a far-off point
on an opposite wall, steely
as a dancer or a fashion model,
their gaze a mooring, a slip knot
to stabilize the vessel.
Instead, they drift, snagged
from the instructor by the tufting hair
of the person in the front of the room,
by the toe that bobs back to the mat
for balance, for the wobbling
of the person between you and the window—
so many pedicures! the elderly
feet Rembrandt might have tried
but with blue French tips
or a hibiscus accent nail.
Then the heating coils of the ceiling,
the piercing lights in their gym cages,
and back to the bodies, the rows
of distracting bodies.
We are here to align them
with our thoughts, these bodies,
But you stare at your own leg
that forms the base of your triangle,
when did it get like that—
branching coral and sea fans
formed of veins, rising to the surface,
the hidden struggles visible?
The eye darts among these ruins
like fishes, sunlit in the depth.
We pause, we breathe, a soughing in and out
Like a wave. We try to ride it,
To let go.

The Natural Spirit of the Gong in Meditation
Nonfiction by Barbara Lee Gray

There is a recording of Earth's magnetic field made some years ago when Voyager took off for a trip through the solar system. This nineteen-minute song of Earth is available through various cymatic and NASA websites. The sounds that emanate from our planet resonate around us in frequencies that we respond to but do not readily hear. This is called the Shuman Resonance and is vital to all life on our planet. It's curious that these tones sound very much like a gong when it is played lightly in the still of the night. Modern society quakes with the crash and din of our industrialized world. Beneath this raucous cacophony of sound, Earth hums its own song that keeps us alive despite the bashing sound and noise pollution. The gong is a respite from this loudness, perhaps to connect us, the essence of our beings, to the frequency of our births. In this healing, we return to our original gifts of creativity, peace, and love.

The gong has been in use for thousands of years. In some societies, the gong was sounded to gather villages together for important announcements. At present, the gong finds its use as a percussion instrument in symphonic bands or rock music; it is often used in some households as a dinner chime. The gong is regularly used in the practice of kundalini yoga, whose benefits encompass the existential entirety of the human being.

Usually at the first session, practitioners of kundalini yoga learn how each set, pose, or meditation balances the sympathetic and parasympathetic nervous systems. The various kriyas, pranayamas and meditations (or sets) increase the parasympathetic response—72,000 nerves—to allow one to accumulate the grit necessary to face the challenges of life. The word, *kundalini*, derives from the *kundal*, or coiled energy at the base of the spine. This energy is coiled three and a half times. This dormant energy is awakened once a person takes on the practice of kundalini yoga.

Many of the meditations of kundalini yoga are in the form of chants that speak to the soul and awaken the body to healing or enlightenment. To begin, a person calls on their "source of infinite creative wisdom... the divine teacher within." This chant awakens and centers the practitioner for a set or a meditation. In addition to the chants that prepare the body, mind, and spirit for a kundalini yoga set, there are chants for healing sickness, chants for psychological balance, chants for peaceful well-being, and so on. Often, these chants and songs are the scheduled meditative activity in a yoga set.

One of these meditations is the gong meditation. To regenerate the parasympathetic system, Yogi Bhajan says that the gong is the best. According to Yogi Bhajan:

> The Gong is the first and last instrument for the human mind, there is only one thing that can supersede and command the human mind, the sound of the Gong. It is the first sound in the universe, the sound that created this universe. It's the basic creative sound. To the mind, the sound of the Gong is like a mother and father that gave it birth. The mind has no power to resist a Gong that is well played.

In kundalini yoga, the mantra of the gong meditation is the sound of the gong, whose waves penetrate every cell of the body. These waves create pressure to relieve the nervous system of any illness by balancing the sympathetic and parasympathetic nervous systems. If the gong is played for eleven minutes or longer, Yogi Bhajan suggests that no food or water be consumed because the gong meditation cleans nerve endings and allows both sympathetic and parasympathetic systems to interact. Any distraction in this process will divert the healing energy of the gong.

I became familiar with the gong after attending several gong baths at a kundalini yoga studio in Nashville and other venues. After a year or so, I found a symphonic gong on sale at an online store. When I got the gong, I immediately played it for people, even though I was a bit clumsy at it. The first gong meditation I played was on New Year's Day for a group at a house party. It was a rather loud and disorganized experience for me. One thing I did, though, is to play patterns and angles along the surface of the gong, triangles, squares, and such. Even at this first meditation, I noticed that certain areas of the gong produce their own unique sound waves.

The more I play the gong, the more sensitive I get to the subtleties of frequency, as well as how sound waves bounce off each other and through each other. The patterns I play on the surface of the gong often resemble the patterns created by musicians who practice cymatics in the laboratory. I don't plan on any particular pattern before a gong meditation, so the patterns just come out of my arms and onto the gong.

No two gong meditation sessions are the same. Each experience has been different, and I believe it is because there is always a different group from one session to another. One reason that I ask for the doors to be locked when we start is that the group in deep meditation would be changed remarkably by the addition of another person or set of vibrations, if you will. As vibrations from the gong dance around, they blend with each other to create new sounds at various points throughout the space above and within the listeners. The sound waves of the gong are mostly out of tune with each other. The result is that along the scale of musical notes, there are an infinite number of combinations in tone or frequency that can be achieved by the gong. Each listener has a unique experience because the vibrations don't collide with each other at the same time, place, or wavelength during the gong meditation. The sounds seem to wash together. The gong meditation is often referred to as a gong bath for this reason.

To put this more simply, each listener has a set of frequencies that resonate only around them due to the chaotic properties of the sound waves coming from the gong. The resulting vibrations from the people who are meditating influence the sound vibrations bouncing around the room, and this lends uniqueness to each experience. Because the sound waves bounce around differently from one person to the other, each set of ears listens in hemi-sync fashion. In a hemi-sync recording, separate sets of frequencies are perceived in each ear, and these frequencies combine to create a unique sound that can only be heard in the mind of the listener. As a result, the experience is also deeply personal for everyone. The patterns I play on the gong bounce and flow around the room and become new patterns in and around the meditation practitioners. As a result, the meditation affects the frequency at which each person in the room vibrates.

Our bodies always vibrate, and these vibrations are measureable in the form of brain waves. Beta brain waves, which resonate between 12Hz and 30Hz, are associated with waking consciousness, logic, and reasoning. We go through our daily routines and express our habits in this state. It is the state in which we are unaware of the self; we focus on objects, thoughts, and feelings. Alpha brain waves, which vibrate between 7.5Hz and 12Hz, are present when we relax our minds with eyes closed or while day-dreaming. Alpha waves influence imagination, visualization, memory, learning, and concentration.

The theta state is the realm of the subconscious mind and vibrates below 7.5 Hz. This is the state we experience as we fall asleep, that chasm between the worlds of dreams and reality. A sense of spiritual connection with the universe, or "Unified Field," can be experienced at theta levels of awareness. Waves of inspiration, creativity, insight, and the mental home of our most deep-seated habits are the essence of theta.

Again, kundalini yoga teaches that the frequencies of the gong resonate with our sympathetic and parasympathetic systems to heal on a deep level of our being. The electric grid of our parasympathetic system is our nervous system. The nervous system is structured to reverberate in the same vibrational state as the Unified Field. John Hagelin, International President of the Global Union of Scientists for Peace, Physics Professor at Maharishi University of Management, shows mathematical tables that illustrate the various degrees of freedom (or movement of vibrations) along the Unified Field in his presentation, *Is Consciousness the Unified Field?*, at the 2011 Science and Non-Duality Conference. This is the vibration of consciousness.

According to Hagelin, the theta is a state of "open monitoring." When people meditate regularly, they connect all parts of their brains. When meditation does not occur, there is random electrical activity, and no connection takes place. The natural harmonics of universal mind are the "sequential emergence of the Unified Field" (Hagelin).

The voice of theta is the silence of the universal mind, and the sound of the gong can help us achieve this state without falling asleep. Ultimately, gamma brain waves (39-100 Hz) are involved in complex mental activity, and a study has shown that advanced Tibetan meditation practitioners produce higher levels of gamma waves both before and during meditation than those who don't practice meditation (*Brain and Health*). Gamma brain waves resonate with the same frequencies as sound waves, and this is the basis for how the sound of the gong affects the vibrations of our minds and bodies.

At the start of the gong meditation, we hold an intention. Intention manifests in the Unified Field, and the Unified Field operates on calculable frequencies. The natural reverberant tones are the elementary particles of light, gravity, electrons, Higgs' spin zero, and so on (Hagelin). These elementary particles flow along the DNA grid from vibrational tones to force, to matter, and they enumerate waves of fundamental consciousness from nothing to activity. Hold an intention and affect the "chaotic, bubbling Unified Field" (Hagelin). Pure consciousness is thought on a very deep level, attainable through meditation and accelerated with the gong. John Hagelin puts it so beautifully when he says that the "vibrational tones are the natural reverberant frequencies of Universal Mind, the music of the absolute. The Unified Field is teeming unmanifest energy, shimmering, infinitely energetic vibrations of erupting, a boiling of the absolute."

At the beginning of the gong bath, the listeners get comfortable and warm since they will be focusing their bodies and minds for over an hour. The sound of the gong lowers the body temperature in some people. This may be because in this level of awareness, the body's energy is focused on the frequencies and vibrations in the sympathetic and parasympathetic systems. At intervals during the meditation, I use a "whale wand" to play the songs of whales along the edge and surface of the gong. According to Yogi Bhajan's instructions, there are three intervals of the gong's crescendo; I follow his protocol and end with a meditative composition so that the group can transition from meditative to waking states.

After the gong meditation is over and the group wakes, people discuss their experiences. It is important for people to talk or listen to others talk so that they can reorient themselves to the more conscious, beta level. As a result of the meditation, many people feel relief from chronic pain, depression, stress, or any combination of distress. The focus of the gong meditation does not have to necessarily center on an ailment or illness. One woman told me that she reworked an idea that she had long forgotten. Another person experienced vivid dreams during the meditation. Almost everyone finds a deeper calm within, relief from anxiety, and reduced cortisol levels in the blood. This reduces inflammation throughout the body.

When we are in places of total silence such as the Badlands in South Dakota, both earthly and universal frequencies are unobstructed so that they can flow through the body more freely and completely. There are few places on earth that have virtually no noise pollution where the earth resonates through the silence. In our busy noise-infested societies, it is difficult to slow down and absorb these waves that flow from the deep recesses of the universe, through Earth, and vibrate within us. We absorb the stressful sounds of the modern world and either pass this negativity on or absorb it in one situation or another. The gong creates an infinite number of sound waves that the body, mind, and spirit can resonate with and absorb. The gong meditation fulfills the need for Earth's natural wave of sound in each of us, as a balm against the barrage of dissonance between us.

Bibliography

Hagelin, John. "Is Consciousness the Unified Field? A Field Theorist's Perspective." Lecture. *Science and Non-Duality*. 19 Jul. 2014. Web. YouTube. 3 Jan. 2016.
Shue, Karen. "The Basics of Brainwaves." *Brain and Health*. n.d. Web. 16 Dec. 2015.

OHM
Poetry by Jessica Ruby Hernandez

Oh sweet surrender of my nose to my toes,
Oh sacred longing to be in Divine Flow,
Oh life-force prana,
enlivening every pose,
oh internal power,
quietly returning home,
ahhh, peaceful stillness:
I have the Yoga Glow!
~~Ohhhhmmm~~

Unrolling the Mat
Nonfiction by Sarah Cunningham, LCSW, CYT

It all began with yoga, when I was brought to my mat, post knee surgery, consumed by depression, lethargy, and weight gain. In a synchronous way that neither she nor I could understand at the time, the instructor handed me my new yoga studio membership card and stated, "Congratulations on taking the first step in changing your life." She had no way of knowing that this profound statement would, in fact, be true.

Like many people, I first fell in love with what yoga did for my body. I was able to shed the weight I had gained and developed muscle tone unlike I had ever had before (note: I was a "gym rat" for years, dreaming of toned biceps and triceps to complement my quickly sagging arm tattoo). I looked and felt great. It would be sometime however before I realized that yoga was so much more than poses.

A therapist by trade, I began to see the parallel between yoga and mental health. When I stepped onto my mat it became a mirror, reflecting back both my outer and inner states. If I ate or drank too much the night before, there it was. If I was emotionally strained, there it was. I began to hear the voice inside. It became louder, clearer, and what I heard, I did not like.

Plagued by anxiety for the majority of my life, I was well aware of the worried and often cruel words that would swim through my head. But, it was on my mat where I learned how to develop a relationship with the pain. Without running away or shutting down, I instead learned how to listen. I hated what I heard so the natural inclination was to shut it down, turn it off, and push it down and away. The mirror was still there, reflecting back the patterns of coping strategies that allowed me to dig deeper into my hole. My true self was buried beneath years of shame and fear of never being good enough.

I wish I could say it was a poetic process: chakras aligned, yoga gods smiling down upon me, life in balance, "OM." What manifested was quite the opposite indeed. The further I explored the more I discovered what was lurking in the shadow of my mind. Like the ripples in a turbulent pond, the chaos at the surface kept me from seeing down into the depths of myself. As I learned through yoga to calm the waters, I hadn't yet learned how to deal with what I would see. My "junk" was there in plain sight. Now what? Clean it up or churn the waters once again and hide what I had seen.

Seeing the junk in the bottom of your pond is like seeing a monster in your closet. Each time, regardless of whether or not the monster was there, you sure as hell would brace yourself for its presence each time you opened the door and switched on the light. There would be no way to ignore my junk, even if I wanted to. I could go into detail about what I saw but that's another story written on another day. It is how I managed those monsters, however, that transformed my yoga practice into something beyond a confrontation of fears. I have learned to breathe, and it is through breath that my life has changed.

With a history of panic attacks, I saw breath as the enemy, scarier than that furry little fucker hiding in the closet. Forced to face my junk, I turned toward the fear, toward the breath, and learned how to take back the control that my fear had robbed me of for far too long. With fluid, audible, *ujjayi* (victorious breath) exhalations, I learned to release the tension in my chest which also released me from the paralyzing grip of my thoughts. In this way, the monster I feared in breathing became my best friend. What I feared had unlocked my freedom.

Plagued by panic attacks when confined to small spaces, I had lost my ability to travel—a loss so profound it pains me even now to think of how significantly the fear had paralyzed me. All of that changed in February of last year, when I booked a thirteen-hour flight to Delhi, India. Equipped with my new yoga tools, and an emergency bottle of Xanax, I boarded the plane. It was one of the scariest moments of my life. The trip, the whole experience, brought my yoga practice from my mat and into my life. I've never been so scared and yet so empowered. Between the waves of fear, I found stillness, calm, and space amidst the thoughts and sensations as they arose.

In India, I learned to ride the waves, breaking a lifelong pattern of trying to fight against them. Yoga is a practice, so I work on this fact every single day. I catch myself treading water, churning up the waves, and emerging like a wet dog, dripping with unnecessary struggle. And yet, I emerge with awareness, looking back into the mirror of my mat toward my reflection of all that I now see.

What I see, yes, sometimes, I still fear, but equipped with my yoga, I look straight ahead into the eyes of my true self, and find I love what I now see. Yoga has taught me that "everything you want in life is on the other side of fear" and that, in fact, I am capable of looking fear in the eye. In this way, my life began, and it all started because I rolled out my mat.

Taking Flight
Poetry by Ariel Bowlin

It takes courage to breathe.

You must have faith in yourself to fill up your lungs
and give your body, mind and spirit
what they crave.

For too long I took for granted the one thing I needed most.
I held it in, waiting for life to get easier.

Even when I did dare to breathe, it was shallow and quiet,
as if I was afraid I didn't deserve it.

Maybe I believed that in order to find balance I should hold back and
be restrained.

Fortunately, asana taught me to reach for more.
Finding balance on the mat helped me to do more and be more.

I had to find myself in that impossible place in space,
teetering on one foot or two hands or ten
fingertips.

Only on that precipitous edge was I finally able to say,
"This is possible."

I can hold this flight.
I can be and do what I dream of.

With each exhale I will shed myself of doubt, expectations and fear.
With each inhale I will imprint my true desire on every cell of my being.

Since breath is necessary to stay balanced,
I am grateful that the demands of balance
Helped me to find my breath.

Choose Happy
Nonfiction by Laura Rose Schwartz

In my 33rd year, during the aftermath of the most transformative experience of my life, my heart was broken open. I now view my life as the time before my heart was open, and the time after. There was a period of healing in between the two, almost like a cocoon preparing me for how to handle the time after, emerging delicate-skinned and hopeful and a completely different person, able to see the world through the lens of open heart.

In the before period, there was no purpose. There was just...life, and a sad life. I grew up never feeling good enough—not smart enough, not pretty enough, not deserving enough of love. Not deserving of anything, really. These feelings were reinforced by a family always expecting me to do well, but never telling me either that I did well or that what I did was good. My father was absent and my mother emotionally detached. I picked up on these behaviors, longing for close friendships and love but never understanding the how. I had friends but I felt outcast and alone, and ugly because no boys seemed romantically interested. If they were, my crippling shyness put an end to any possibilities of butterflies and first kisses. And then the feelings of loneliness, and otherness, and "outsiderness" became a self-fulfilling prophecy—I did not feel enough because I didn't have love, and I didn't have love because I didn't feel enough.

I allowed my lack of confidence to mar relationships, always seeking reassurance, but never believing it when received. When I began to date, the men I met used my anxiety and fear to make me feel even less than I already did. I believed them when they told me I was the destroyer of lives, that all bad in the relationships was my fault, that the hell they subjected me to, the cruelty—emotional and mental especially, but not only—was because I made them angry. Whereas, in fact, I was just a girl, afraid to use her voice—afraid to protest, afraid to ask for help, afraid to ask for love, afraid to say she'd had enough and leave. So I began to crave the darkness, escape, sleep. And, I became destructive towards myself in order to find the nothingness. It became more important than anything. That was my life in the before.

They say—whoever the wise sages are who pervade our general colloquial wisdom—that your heart must break before it opens. I kept feeling like there was no more hurt that I could endure, that each down must be the worst it could get. But, how many times must a heart break before it is past repair, nonfunctional? I became obsessed with my own sadness, my story of tragedy. At a certain point, I knew that I had to make a choice, that I could continue to seek out darkness and fade away, or I could try, one more time, to live again. So, I sought help, and the question that made me pause and gave me hope was, "What in my life made me want to feel?" And, the answer to that pause and question was yoga.

I am an impulsive person by nature. I believe this stems from an inability to trust my decisions. I have never felt capable of being an adult, regardless of any achievements or success or evidence to the contrary. Once the question was asked and answered, I decided on impulse to become a yoga teacher. Then, I decided to go to a foreign land and become one.

That process, the month long immersion into the depths of me certainly had a great impact. Yet, perhaps what saved me more than anything else, was being loved by a group of strangers who became friends, who cherished me for who I was, just as I was. This overwhelming love pushed me past my breaking point. I didn't know what to do in the "real" world once the training was over. And so, I almost destroyed myself. But that is the origin story of the new creature I have become.

But

my point now is

the light that I was shown, the love of me, with no strings and no demands, the confidence I had learned to have in myself as a teacher, was a whisper of hope that I followed out of the darkness. I no longer wanted to be asleep. An almost primal drive pushed me to fight to live, to crawl out of the hole I thought that I was trapped inside.

The fact that I made that choice, that I valued myself to claw out of that deep dark well of sadness...that was the beginning of everything. I now feel that I am evolving into a creature of strength and love. The old cobwebs of doubt and dark still exist, but mostly I am able to brush them aside. "Choose happy" has become my mantra. That may sound trite, but that mindset helps me, lets me, and reminds me to get through whatever I must face. I am cracked and broken, and I have stories and nightmares and tragedies that few know. Yet, I am strong, beautiful, courageous, brave, and happy. I am enough. That I finally feel love for myself...that is the most beautiful feeling I have ever experienced.

Be.Live.
Poetry by Jasmin Serina

Searching for truth
Thundering thought

Darkness evolve
Problems to solve

Quiet mind
Be mine

Believe

Be.Live.

Reflection
Nonfiction by Clarissa Thompson

My teacher closed the yoga class by asking the students to focus our energy in our heart chakra, and the color was a deep, emerald green—I felt the energy center, the pure and deep space that exists in the heart, for the first time in my adult life. That moment offered a glimpse of the power that exists in our own bodies—this was the hook. After that class, I craved more understanding and wanted to experience that openness and warmth again. I wanted the ability to tap into the energy centers and feel what was going on inside the body.

I sought out workshops, books, videos, stories about breath, energy, yoga, and meditation. I began meditating as part of a group that would meet at the studio space. I felt the sensations of group energy, when we would chant together and meditate together. I started to understand, at least partially, that my body, mind, and spirit were all connected, and not just because they were mine, but because they were all part of a larger force—the breath force, the life force, the force of nature.

Fast forward several years and many life-changing experiences later, it was January 2015, and I was at work when I received a text from my mom that my grandma was taken to the hospital in the night. My grandma had been in rehabilitation center after a fall that resulted in a broken hip. At the hospital, Grandma was unresponsive. Mom was going to the hospital which was a ninety-mile drive, and it was the middle of winter. Later that day, I booked a flight when I knew Grandma's condition wasn't getting any better. I spent the next few days with my family. Grandma was moved back to the nursing facility where she was previously living during her rehabilitation. They would care for her until the end.

It was in these last few hours with Grandma that I noticed the feeling, the feeling around my heart, and it was like my whole inside was glowing, a deep emerald green. I sat with Grandma, holding her hand as her body began to shut down. In those last few hours, she was struggling to fight. Her body was struggling to maintain its life force, and it was trying to keep the breath. When I said my goodbye, I kissed her forehead and held her head in my hands just for a moment, doing all I could to give her my peaceful and loving energy so that she would not be in pain. For a brief moment, our eyes met and I knew that she was aware of my presence. That was the last time I would look into her eyes.

The thought of Grandma still brings tears to my eyes, and while her passing is still very sad for me, it was that moment, that split second in time when we connected in this realm for the last time, that fulfills me. Her energy and mine, her spirit and my spirit, sparked off of one another. In the final moments of her life, I think she knew that deep connection, the one that we all strive for while we are living—to feel that spark of energy.

Just less than a year later, I found myself in India, studying at the K Pattahbi Jois Ashtanga Yoga Institute for the month of December. I was surrounded by devoted practitioners, people who had been traveling to India for many years to study and learn from the guru. While in India, I experienced some of the most intense feelings of loneliness and feelings of struggle, as I began to question what I was doing with my life, with my gifts, passions, and talents. Was I really utilizing them to the best of their ability and making the most of my life, or did I just exist day-to-day, too afraid to make the leap?

My experience in India tore me down to my bare minimum, as I felt lost and confused about my path, my identity, and what to do next. In the years that I have practiced yoga, it has transformed who I am— helping me to remove the layers of identity placed on me by my past and has given me the confidence to embrace the person I am without the added layers of so-called protection. I find that when I talk about these real moments with friends and students, and share them via my social networks, people respond with sincerity. I think more people are searching for a way to shed the societal standards of what it means to be "normal" as well as the expectations on happiness and success.

Yoga has taught me to become more in-tune with my whole body, to notice when something doesn't feel right, and to trust my gut. It has also taught me to be more trusting and open to new possibilities and to realize the difference between fear and danger. To be able to tap into the energy stream that connects us all and feel the vibrations of the universe in each step, in each living thing, and moment in time is a true gift. It's the feeling I got the night of my first class, the feeling Grandma and I shared before she passed, and the feelings I struggled to sort through in India. And now, as I write about it, I find that I am able to sit and process those emotions and find the beauty in each moment of struggle.

Open-Hearted
Poetry by Jessica Ruby Hernandez

Empty
vacio
I am a "vaso",
a vessel
for light to enter,
move through me
move me.
Speak to me, Great One,
speak *through* me.
I am open,
receptive,
my antennae are out.
the door to my heart is open;
come on in,
I'll make you some tea.

Author's Notes:
Vacio means "empty" in Spanish
Vaso means "drinking glass" in Spanish

Yoga—a forever faithful relationship that endures the ebb and flow of life
Nonfiction by Leslie Storms, RN, MSN, E-RYT 500

It concerns itself not of the common place thoughts: (I have a headache, I am too old, and my hip is aching).

Yoga has but one simple request: Please, practice with love and sincerity of the heart. Each and every day, yoga gracefully invites one to explore and brush upon those meaningful questions, such as: "Am I deeply connecting with my own sense of authenticity?"

Yoga has such a special way of expressing itself. It is a loving opportunity to know thyself. It has the power to penetrate and transform weakness into strength and struggle into liberation.

That seedling of surrender hides within the breath. It is a sacred invitation to look softly inside, to peel back the layers of fear and suffering, and sincerely to listen from the heart and connect to the Divine. That tender opening is revealed there amongst the silent spaces, patiently waiting between the inhalation and exhalation.

This expansive presence unwaveringly cradles the truth of who we are. And unbeknownst to most, anyone with a willing heart will surprisingly realize the truth simply through the devotion and practice of yoga.

At first, it is most often summoned as a feeling or a taste—a tiny taste of the illusions that keep one hidden from the truth (of who we are). This experience sustains the beginning yogi, as the desire and quest for just one more taste catapults the seeker onward.

The quiet internal thoughts begin to pass: What gives of this yoga? Where did that sweetness come from? Who offered that taste of freedom to me?

The craving for that indescribable feeling ignites a desire for more— the feeling of being fully alive, free from the constant perpetual restraints of the mind. But what one does not know as a novice is that Spirit is and was always present.

You just finally surrendered: you became quiet in the physical body, you released expectations, and you opened your heart to listening.

You stepped into silence and in that silence you discovered a union with grace. You tasted your purest potential.

•

I Am Yoga
Poetry by Jessica Ruby Hernandez

I am yoga.
I am the breath that flows in,
that pauses, sometimes catches in my throat,
and slowly flows out.
I am the sweet surrender to my higher self.
I am messy, stubborn ego.
I am control and
I am control relinquished.
I am my shadow,
And I am my light.
I am the unknown outcome, whether
my pose is beautiful/perfect/social media worthy,
or not.
Does it matter?
I am the voice inside my head
in Goddess pose.
Does this voice cheer me on,
or tell me to quit?
It has done both.
I am the squirm and the grimace
of my face as the mental yoga ensues.
I am Hanuman's giant leap—
well, not yet,
maybe next year.
I am the grace. I am the wild thing.
I am crumpled up in a ball in child's pose,
crying profusely.
I am the sweet victory of
destroying my mental barriers.
I am the devastated failure
at taming my monkey-mind.
I am perfectly balanced on one foot,
and I am a tree in a hurricane.
I am vulnerable courage.
Exposing my Self to myself.

Every. Damn. Day.
I am awkward.
I am awakened.
My mind is captivated by my breath
Most days.
I am yoga.

I Am
Nonfiction by Jessica Gibbs

I am. These are two simple words to some people. They are possibly the two hardest words for me, especially when followed by another word. Yet, I awake each morning and utter these very words while staring into my eyes in the mirror. Some days my eyes appear shiny and deep green, the color of the pines. Other days, they are clouded by the film of tears, dull blue, and I want nothing more than to look away. Though, I don't. I carry on and know the feelings will pass. I understand, too, that I am much further along the road of self love than when I started.

***

I didn't want to do part of the social media challenge. It seemed so simple, to record myself saying, "I am..." along with a laundry list of good qualities. All I had were five: kind, patient, loving, fun, and funny. That's it. And to be honest, I had only come up with the words *kind* and *patient*. The other three I got from frequent comments by other people on my social media sites. The thought crossed my mind more than once that it was quite sad how I could not rapidly come up with more nice qualities about myself. Then, the negative cycle started. My thoughts would spin out of control and go down the dark path of words from the past that I had tried to block out. These words were not holding an ounce of truth, but I chose to believe them anyway.

"Stupid whore."

"Dumb."

"Slut."

"Bitch."

"I don't love you. You don't deserve to be loved."

For the first four negatives, I could rationalize that they were not true. The last phrase closed my heart, even though it was said more than a decade ago. And although I had much love to give to the world, I had none for myself and continued to choose to punish myself, believing that I was not worthy of love. It did not matter how hard I tried—the awards I won, the degrees I obtained, the level of physical strength and bravery I displayed—none of it was enough. I was not enough. I would never be enough.

This reason, of not being enough, was the exact reason I chose to do the yoga challenge. So, I put my phone's camera in the reverse mode and tried to look myself in the eyes. Instantly, my eyes darted away. I felt the fluttering of one hundred moths come into my chest, as my throat went tight and my eyes filled with hot tears. Still, I brought my eyes back to center, focusing first on my chin, then my nose, and finally meeting my gaze on the small screen. I saw dark circles hanging under dull, blue eyes and a crooked nose below them. I saw teeth that weren't white enough, even though they shone in pictures and people complimented them frequently. However, I held my gaze, eyes filling with tears and hit the record button on my phone.

"I am kind."

"I am patient."

"I am loving."

"I am fun."

"I am funny."

"I am anxious."

Crap. I didn't mean to say that. Why did the word *anxious* come out? I was supposed to say positive qualities, and I could not even do that.

Again, I felt a bit sad after watching other challenge participants post their videos. I could see confidence beginning to shine in their eyes, yet I still had trouble meeting my own.

I went to my yoga mat feeling defeated. I practiced anyway, trying to lose myself through the poses of an online class. I was trying to let go of not being able to complete the challenge of self love the way I had envisioned.

Time passed. Asanas passed, too. I practiced with a vengeance, trying to run away from myself and ignoring the feelings the challenge had brought up. I began to land *eka pada bakasana* (one-legged crane pose). I performed in an aerial show. I became the "favorite" at my job. But none of it was enough.

My marriage was still falling apart, which made me feel even more like a failure and more unloved. Out of all the successes in my life, if I couldn't have a successful marriage, then I must not be worthy of love. I completed more asanas and more activities to fill the time and ignore these feelings.

Until, I could no longer ignore the feelings. I felt on edge. Tears were just a breath away from threatening to spill over the corners of my eyes. My chest felt tight. I'd had a terrible case of bronchitis for six months and had to stop strenuous activity, lest I would end up wheezing on the floor. This feeling was how closed my heart had become, wrapped tightly in layers of rope until I could barely squeeze a breath in or out of my body without a hacking cough, or crying. I tried to deny my bundled heart, but the feelings were there, eking out from time to time like water seeping through cracks and finding its way to the ground.

I had reached my rock bottom.

I made the decision. Something must change. And with that decision, I made three important shifts in my practice and my life—two on the mat and one off the mat.

On the mat, I began practicing heart openers and started meditating after reading about it and its effects on people. The third change was insisting my husband go to marriage counseling with me. I thought that if I fixed "us," then "I" would be fixed. I was naïve, I suppose, as I had no idea of the journey about to begin.

The first counseling session was a getting acquainted session. Not much changed. I liked the therapist and related to her instantly. My husband and I went home with some small homework tasks, and life crept along. I kept up with my physical yoga practice, sometimes for two or three hours until 1 a.m. By then, I was too tired to notice my sad heart in its cage. Asanas are endless. I felt that I would never master them, and I would never be enough, so I kept trying to get better and better—to maintain balance in *pincha mayurasana* (feathered peacock pose), to flip my grip in *dhanurasana* (bow pose), and to be flat on the floor in *hanumanasana* (monkey pose, also known as splits). I foolishly tried to make the poses enough to ignore my heart.

I still meditated once a week and started having brief seconds of peace before the madness of my thoughts went galloping around my brain's racetrack again. I thought maybe the meditation would help calm the anxiety I felt about not being enough.

As counseling sessions added up, old wounds surfaced. I cried more and more with each session. After each one, I went to my mat with puffy eyes and a stinging face from where the tears had flowed. I finished each practice feeling exhausted, skipping *savasana*, and thinking I would meditate another night. I was not ready to face my heart.

This pattern continued until the day that the racetrack horses of my thoughts came to a tumbling halt during a counseling session. My counselor had been harping on this lesson for several weeks. It finally hit home.

"You are enough. You are *so* enough," she said.

I heard a droplet of truth in those words. My heart began to flutter through the ropes that I had tied around it. That same week, my counselor gave me homework. It was the same activity from the challenge several months prior. I had to list ten positive qualities about myself.

I had to look in the mirror every day for a week and say, "I am _____."

I thought, "I am screwed."

I still couldn't come up with ten words. I used the five from before and again added a few more that I had seen other people use to describe me on social media. But the fierceness and conviction of her words to describe me as "enough" caused me to tip my head to the side and ponder my worth. In that moment, I thought, "I'm doing this. I am going to do this self-love thing."

That evening, I went home, found a dry erase marker, and wrote the words on the left-hand side of my mirror in purple, scrawling handwriting.

Kind

Patient

Loving

Caring

Fun

Funny

Adventurous

Brave

Strong

Badass

And then, almost as an afterthought, I added the phrase "I am enough" at the bottom of the mirror and drew a lopsided heart beside it. I nodded to myself in the mirror and then went to bed in what had become my room, while my husband slept in his room. The next day, my morning mantras would begin.

I awoke groggy, hitting the snooze button two times, and then my eyes flew open as I remembered the mantras. I jumped out of the bed, flipped on the lights in the bathroom, and grabbed the edge of the bathroom counter. I lifted my eyes to meet my reflection's gaze in the mirror.

"I. . ."

"I. . ."

My eyes felt hot with tears and shame. Why couldn't I do this simple thing? I slammed one hand on the counter, determined to finish.

"I am kind."

"I am patient."

"I am loving."

Pause. I couldn't remember any more qualities and had to look to my left at my list.

Shit.

Deep breath in and out.

"I am caring."

"I am fun."

"I am funny."

"I am adventurous."

Pause. Again, I could not remember any more positive words. My eyes dropped down, focusing on the stopper in the sink, thinking how I needed to clean the whole apartment. My eyes shifted back to the left, and I began again.

"I am brave."

"I am strong."

"I am a badass."

"And I am enough."

I said these eleven phrases. I made it to the end, tears streaming down my face. I leaned my back against the wall, slid to a squat on the floor, buried my head into my knees, and began to cry. My chest shuddered with sobs and shallow breaths. I realized that I would be late to work, so I heaved myself up from the floor, hurriedly got dressed and ready for work, and left the mantras behind.

This routine of morning mantras, meditation, and my physical yoga practice continued for several weeks. I had started repeating the mantra "I am enough" during each meditation and at the end of my morning mantras, which to my surprise, became easier on some days. I did not cry every morning when saying the mantras. I began to memorize the words and feel them vibrate through my lips with meaning.

Counseling sessions also continued, but my husband stopped attending shortly after our fifth wedding anniversary. It seemed ironic to me because five is my "lucky number," yet I could not seem to turn the marriage around after five years of practice. I felt a sense of failure, shame weighing heavily on my heart, winding another coil around it and making it harder to feel what my heart wanted.

Since my husband stopped going to counseling, the sessions now became partly about our marriage and mostly about me. I felt my bound heart was under the microscope and twitching. I felt it pulsing through the ropes, beating a bit faster in anticipation as it knew something was about to happen.

I started journaling daily at the recommendation of my counselor. It was a habit I practiced on and off again throughout the years. It felt good to put the pen to the paper, to scratch out my thoughts, fears and hopes. I wrote at least three pages a day in a 99-cent spiral-bound notebook. I ended each day by writing one of my mantras ten times on the last ten lines of the third page, giving life to the words. This lent the words a sense of permanency.

The spoken mantras became easier with each morning that passed. I could speak these phrases without tears most days and without looking at the list. I had even added a couple words of my own along with a few from social media: amazing, creative, hard-working, and dedicated. My heart continued to race each morning just before saying these words, but I had committed to the journey.

I felt the shift in my physical yoga practice too, and began craving heart openers. I decided that I was ready to try to grab my ankles in *dwi pada viparita dandasana* (two-legged inverted staff pose). I carefully worked my body into the pose after my practice. I pushed my head between my arms, trying to expand and puff out my heart. Then, I felt a ripping sensation down my sternum and a rush of exhilaration. I came out of the pose feeling a bit disoriented, thinking I had broken or injured something. To my surprise, nothing in my physical body had changed. I took savasana in a state of shock.

Somehow, a knife had sliced through the top layers of rope around my heart. I felt it expanding with each "lub-dub" pounding between my chest and my mat, the sound roaring in my ears.

I awoke the next day and said my morning mantras, running quickly through the list. My voice was a bit stronger and my eyes never wavered from the reflection in the mirror. I felt the change coming, and with it, fear. Doubt. Shame. But also, a tiny voice reminded me...

"I am strong."

"I am brave."

"I am enough."

The voice continued to get louder. I heard it ask for a divorce. And after the shock of that moment, of hearing my voice say the words to free me, the weight of the ropes around my heart uncoiled. My heart flew madly around the perimeter of my chest, not having tasted flight for over a decade, but still trapped within the confines of my ribs. For that time, it was enough. I was enough on that day. I had myself again. And I was enough.

***

As the 4th of July approaches this year, it reminds me of that period of time in my life. That was a time when I was just beginning to see my strength, the glimmer of me, and the fragments of me coming back together. I remember watching fireworks through the old apartment's window, squeezing myself between towers of packed boxes to watch the bursts of light through teary eyes.

My physical practice of asanas has continued, but it has gotten softer around the edges. I no longer need a perfect practice to justify my self worth. I no longer need to "get" a pose. I did need that type of practice for a time, and it was an important step during the journey. Yet, now my yoga path has become more creative. I use it as a tool to listen to myself and, in turn, I am better able to hear my heart and be of service to others. Some days are still filled with a strenuous physical practice until one in the morning. Other days, I might cry in pigeon pose. I've learned to listen to my body and my heart, and to stop myself when I start trying to prove something to myself—whether on the mat or off the mat. I am enough without that asana. I am also enough without another person.

My life is all still very much a work-in-progress. I still wake every morning and tell myself at least ten positive qualities and end with the phrase, "And I am enough." I've also added, "Hi, Jessica. You are beautiful, and I love you. I love all of you." These words are still written in purple marker on my apartment mirror. I still meditate every day, some days with racing thoughts and other days seeing colors and shapes.

I would be lying if I said any of the above was easy. It isn't. It is a process. If anything, it is harder because now I am more aware. I still have days where I fall into and experience old patterns of using relationships or other people to justify my self worth. The difference is that now, I'm able to recognize that pattern and re-direct. I often take time alone to reflect and get myself back on track with what my counselor calls "self care."

Yoga—the mantras, the asanas, the breath, and the meditation—all of it has helped to heal me and continues to heal me. It has finally helped me to realize that I am enough. Just as I am. And, I am still working toward a consistent stance, believing I am worthy of love, not only from others, but more importantly, from myself.

I continue on this journey of self-love in order to bring more love to the world around me *and* to myself. I continue to practice yoga, to meditate, and to listen to my heart. I continue to say the morning mantras because I am enough.

I am *so* enough.

And, I am definitely worth it.

Doing Yoga with James Taylor
Poetry by C.T. Kern

Wednesday, twenty minutes after the hour
and we're past the initial chatting and stretching
in the half-lit back room where muted
we hear the cadenced warnings
from the cardio circuit that warn
Thirty seconds, you have thirty seconds,
as though it's a memento mori and not
the incentive to pedal faster.
We're looking at the sliding doors
for the teacher, waiting, for the way
she enters, for the way she hurries
without rushing, as the Dalai Lama
might walk if he were about to miss a plane,
if the Dalai Lama had frizzy red hair.
We're already looking at the woman
in the front row, to see if she'll start us
in Mountain, swooping our hands
to the caged lights and industrial tubing.
But in she comes, our teacher,
with her denim bag and mat, even
her apologies calm, like someone
used to forgiving. And then her CD
is missing, so instead of strings
and flutes, we have Fire and Rain,
our fingers pulling
to the sky, against all our bulk
and stiffness and worries,
with Carolina on our minds.

Cultivate
Nonfiction by Laura Rose Schwartz

No one tells a baby how to be happy. We know that babies intrinsically know how to be happy. And, they show us their happiness, sadness, fear, and love both spontaneously and tenderly. Then, as the baby becomes a child, other voices—the voices of parents, friends, partners, society—start to take over and tell them what is important, what is right or wrong, what to value. Some of this is part of being alive and necessary. In so many other ways, it causes us to turn off our true voice, to question our dreams, and, ultimately, to question our worth. We slowly start to lose the innate ability to believe in ourselves.

I lost my inner child for a long time and questioned everything I did. I believed that I was broken and beyond hope. Then, I found yoga, which encourages the inquiry into the self. Within that, I began to heal and to cultivate my voice, my belief in myself, and my abilities. I cultivate pride and gratitude for my strengths, and compassion for my weaknesses. My mat is the soil upon which I cultivate a space where I love myself, where the voice that I had once buried so deeply is allowed to grow and thrive, and where the seeds of opportunity that have always been within are manifested.

Home
Poetry by J. Ray

I find calmness,
though the rest of the world continues to hurry by.
With each deep inhale,
the universe becomes a part of me.
With each exhale,
I become a part of it.

Slowly, focused, guided by my breath, I begin to move.
Every line carefully created,
Every movement fluidly connected.
Never pulled back to my surroundings,
Never rushed by deadlines.
Simply allowing myself to be.

To bend, contract, open, evolve, surrender,
To extend not only my body but my soul.
There is no judgment, comparing, competition,
It has all been replaced with stillness of the mind, releasing of
emotions, and tears mixed with sweat pooling upon the top of my mat.

Every shift of my body,
Accompanied by a shift of my mind.
Pain, anguish, sorrow,
Flowing away from my body.
Love, happiness, gratitude,
Finding its way back into my heart.

Every nerve ignited,
Every sense heightened.
I am home.

To Find My Breath
Nonfiction by Summer Breeze Flowers

Life is filled with so many stressors and ups and downs that we often find ourselves stuck in the chaos crashing down while trying to rush our way through it all. Life can become involuntary very quickly, and we can just "go through the motions" at any given time. When we slow ourselves down, become aware of the now, of the moment we are experiencing, then we can begin to enjoy and savor each moment. In order to slow ourselves down, we must learn to find deep breath. This may seem simple, considering breathing is something we do involuntarily, and we do it all the time. However, when we actively make breathing voluntary, we feel the change of being aware of our breath and aware of the rise and fall in our diaphragms each time we breathe.

Babies breathe with their bellies; this is the best way to connect ourselves and to ground our bodies and minds. When life consumes us or something tragic happens, we can so easily lose control because we have lost our connection with healthy breath. It takes effort to reach inside and feel the moment, but when we do, we can find what we are truly capable of experiencing to the fullest.

I told myself, "You're not good enough" so many times that I have believed it. The very fear of failure and not being good enough would stop me from doing so many activities. As I grew older, I began to realize that I was capable of more than I knew. I was surprised when I was successful. I learned there were too many ways that I had allowed myself to be held back by fear—fear of what others might think and fear of what I would think. There was always fear, every time I felt hesitation and resistance.

Then, I began yoga. I pushed myself beyond the "limits" I had set for myself. I began succeeding and doing what I wouldn't have even tried before yoga. I participated in a Bikram yoga 60-day challenge when I learned that if I didn't understand how to breathe in the moment, then I would never make it through these sixty days. I had too much talk in my head. I had too many, "what-will-they-think, I can'ts, and what ifs," going on in my head during each class. These doubts made me think about running away, about not having enough air, and about all sorts of panic. I learned to reach inside myself and find my breath, and there I finally found stillness. I learned that the rise and fall of my breath had a purpose. Through this awareness of breathing, I found courage, and I discovered confidence as I learned my true ability.

There have been many moments that have taken my breath away, making it feel as if there is not enough air to breathe and receive. I have felt as if my heart has been so full of grief and sorrow that it felt as if I could not gasp enough air into my lungs to breathe. In those times, I have rediscovered my breath. Just when I thought I had lost it, I was able to go inside myself and remind myself that I did have enough breath in my lungs and that everything was okay.

Pain and sadness translate in various ways to our brains. Usually, our brains send alerts and danger signals because pain causes the human body to be in distress. We can experience physical pain from emotional sadness. When no one was there in times of panic during my past to remind me that I was enough and that I would make it through the moment, I had to reach within myself and find the strength that I never knew existed. I had to be the person who talks my own self out of the sad, anxious, painful feelings and who restores my own breath and calmness. I couldn't just tell myself something I didn't believe as a quick remedy—no, I had to believe and know it as truth. I needed to *know* that I could breathe and get through whatever was passing in the moment.

When I was pregnant with my second child, I would awaken in the middle of the night in panic attacks, gasping to breathe as my heart beat quickly and mind raced with thoughts. I allowed the racing, gasping panic to continue. *Was I good enough? Could I really do this? Would I be able to be a good mom?* The fears and negative thoughts felt endless. So many images of fear and failure overtook me that it was difficult to breathe. The first time this happened I was stricken with more fear than ever before, and I was desperately afraid! I wondered, *what is this feeling, this episode, I am having?* It was something very new to me, yet felt very real.

I remember sitting in the dark trying to find my breath in between the tears, and when I first found some bit of strength inside me, it was then that I told myself I could control my breath, and that I would be able to get through the fears. Patiently, I slowed my breath down, which slowed my heartbeat. I reminded myself of the mantra I would use in the hot room in Bikram yoga class. This mantra helped me every time I felt as if I couldn't breathe. I would tell myself, "Restore, rejuvenate, replenish." With each rise and fall of my chest and stomach, I reminded myself that I had all the breath I needed. Soon, I calmed down enough to go to sleep. I survived the feeling.

There are still moments when life grabs me so quickly that I cannot prepare for the taking of my breath away. During those moments, I have to reach inside myself once again and remember that I have the strength and the breath to get through this moment. I have learned that life will take unexpected turns and paths that I did not anticipate. Many of these turns and path changes will cause me to doubt myself and to lose my breath in the moment. When that happens, it is important to go back to the basics, to the rise and the fall in my stomach as my lungs fill with air and my brain fills with oxygen, and then, I begin to discover and cultivate a state of calm.

I do not have power or control over all I want during my lifetime, but I do have the power to control my breath. Through conscious breathing, I have learned to create stillness, calmness, and acceptance of the moment that is occurring. The fear can dissipate if I remind myself to breathe.

My lungs and heart will automatically work together to pump blood and oxygen throughout the body, yet they will not automatically calm me unless I am aware with intent. I must actively stop and find my breath or I will feel at a loss for it during fear. Breathing is actually voluntary too, and to have intent is something that has developed through my awareness.

Life will not always go the way I want and plan. When this happens, I cannot just give up, and it is even more important in times like these that I trust in the path presented to me. Our life paths are unknown and unplanned, and this makes it feel scary, to some people. If we trust ourselves and know everything will be all right, then we can work toward peace in the present moment. Happiness and acceptance are inner paths we must create in order to experience them in life. We make choices about which qualities to develop with intent, and we must also learn to accept in order to allow ourselves to survive.

The Moment
Poetry by Clarissa Thompson

It's the moment between the breaths,
The moment between the flexed muscles,
The stretching ligament,
The moment when anything is possible.

It's the moment before you lock your gaze,
Before the smile
Or a nervous expression
Spreads across your face.

This moment when anything is possible.
Anything.
Anything.
Anything.

Could this moment hold the answer?
Is it the universe finally giving in to your plea?
And, are you ready for it?
Are you ready for this moment?

Now...
...Watch
...Listen
...Breathe.

The breath starts.
You inhale,
Breath sliding into your lungs,
Filling your body with fresh air.

Each cell in your body soaks in the goodness,
Lighting up with joy.
You find yourself in the moment.
Now, will you let it be?

To exist in the moment is to exist in the unknown,
To accept the uncertain,
And relish in the empty space,
The space where anything can be created.

Creating "The_Amazing_Arielle"
Nonfiction by Arielle Witt-Foreman

I have a story to tell, yet I question how to tell it. Opening up is a struggle when we want to share and aren't certain or confident about how to do that, especially when our stories make us uncomfortable and we strive not to make others feel that way.

As I get older, it seems to get more difficult to talk about myself. I have participated in the Instagram Yoga Community for around two years now, and even though I know I am not judged, sharing my story is still a struggle.

Like many, I have always wanted to figure out a way to share my "whole" story without feeling judged, and this book has provided the way. My story does not involve a triumph of asanas, but rather a triumph of the self. There is no specific beginning to my journey, but I definitely feel like my life began again around the time that I started practicing yoga.

I found yoga in July of 2013 when my daughter was nine-weeks-old. My doctor suggested a series of low-impact stretches to help my body heal after an emergency C-section. I struggled with the stretches, and I was also very lonely living in a new area with a newborn. I downloaded the Instagram app to my phone in August of 2013 and followed a few people from my Facebook page. One of those people was a girl named Abby with whom I had gone to high school. As I scrolled through her profile, I saw her posting yoga photos for a yoga challenge hosted by @fitqueenirene. What struck me about Abby's photos was her smile. She truly looked happy while she was practicing yoga. I wanted to know the same joy in my life.

I didn't really know what in the world I was doing when I first started practicing yoga. Connecting with others through Instagram allowed me to explore books, videos, and blogs that I found helpful in becoming comfortable with my practice.

The most notable part of my journey has been the transformation of my inner self. As I have practiced yoga and meditated, I have been able to become comfortable with my own company once again. Before yoga, I suffered from anxiety and depression. I used prescription medications to treat these ailments, which eventually led to drug addiction. Using drugs allowed me to escape from the insecurities and pains that plagued me.

Yoga has provided a new way to replace the old addictions. It reminds me not to escape and avoid my mind as drugs once did. Yoga allows me to dive in and discover my dreams and potential. It has shown a way for me to find confidence through postures and apply that confidence to other aspects of my life.

I have watched my growth in several ways, both with my jobs and the decision to pursue hosting my own Instagram yoga challenge series. This creation on Instagram was profound for me in many ways, as I once was an approval addict, too. Putting myself out there on Instagram as @The_Amazing_Arielle has been a way for me to step out of my box and allow people to see me for who I am now.

It has been difficult for me to accept myself as an inspiration to others, particularly those yogis who participate in the challenge on Instagram. As someone who sought approval, I used to enjoy all types of attention, and, for a time, most of the attention I entertained was negative. As I have progressed into a more positive type of life through yoga and meditation, I still attract attention, but it is all through yoga and healthy living. I struggle with accepting that I can be a positive force and beacon to others. Through the journey of hosting four yoga challenges, I have enjoyed the opportunity to communicate with others who have felt transformed by participating. That was one of my goals for creating my yoga challenges.

Yoga has also taught me about balance not only on the mat, but in my life as well. I have dreams for myself that are gigantic, and yoga has helped me to slow down and find ways to manage my time so that I can determine how to accomplish the goals that I set.

Most importantly to my yoga journey, I have learned the power of breathing. Before yoga, I was a cigarette smoker. Through the practice of deep breaths during meditation, I have been able to quit smoking by replacing the inhalation with pure oxygen instead of addictive toxins. The same feeling develops in me with inversions. The feeling of floating is similar to how I felt after I used certain drugs. As I have continued my practice, the connection to addiction has lessened greatly. My initial yoga connection helped me to overcome my former craving and dark mental state.

Anyone has the power to breathe through and pull themselves out of a mindset that causes unhappiness. I have discovered that the power of how I view myself will manifest in how others see me. Yoga helps me to be confident in my story, to rise above fear, and to find personal strength.

Two Friends
Nonfiction by Laura Swan Pollard

I was brought up to believe that two things in life are certain: death and taxes. What a demoralizing outlook to give a ten-year-old. Of course, life is difficult, but it's also miraculous and rather wonderful.

While I accept that taxes and death are inevitable parts of life, this summation of existence is negative. Taxes and death don't speak of life, but rather the opposite, a lack of life and living.

If we are talking about the certainties of life, then we should refer to the breath and the ground. Without both of these, there is no life. There is no better way to know that we are alive than to feel the breath in our lungs and the ground beneath our feet. When we tune in to our breath and the ground supporting us, we feel safe and held, as though we have two constant friends.

Ellen Lee, Chair of the Independent Yoga network, introduced these life certainties to me as two friends, our constant companions in life. Her description resonated profoundly with me, and I was struck by the simplicity, yet coherence of this perspective.

My yoga practice always begins by tuning in to the ground and the breath. Whether in *savasana* (corpse pose) or *padmasana* (lotus pose), I start by feeling the parts of my body which are in contact with the ground. I notice how the ground supports my body, and I allow myself to be held. It draws my attention down, away from my head, into my body and helps me to connect with the earth. I observe my breath. Noticing the sensation as air passes in and out through my nostrils, I follow the breath into my chest, observing where and how the air travels. This routine establishes my approach to my practice. I'm out of my head and attuned to my body. Throughout my practice I return to these safe places of ground and breath. Before moving through standing postures, I spend time in Tadasana (mountain pose), feeling all parts of my feet in contact with the ground, focusing on its support. I take time to observe the breath. Paying attention to my two friends in every pose helps me to find freedom and stability, and it completely stills and comforts my mind.

Every day, I come back to the breath and the ground. Both are concrete, ever-present reminders that I am alive and everything is okay. Any time I feel unsettled or anxious, I connect with the ground and the breath and know that I have all that I need. It's so simple but so powerful. It reminds me to be grateful for this life and to live it.

I hope to pass on this ethos to my children as I believe gratitude is the key to happiness. This is the message I will give my children: Two things in life are certain—the breath and the ground.

Lost and Found
Nonfiction by Brittany Hoogenboom

There was once a little girl who was lost. She was lost in limbo on the path to nowhere, caught up with weak people, and doing unhealthy things. She made choices she promised her mother she would never make. She took the happiness from others, something she promised herself she would never take.

There was once a little girl who was fueled by hate. She was angry and violent. She lived through sex and drugs. She used sex and drugs to cover up the burning pain in the center of her soul. She was looking for something to fill a void, a hole.

There was once a little girl who lost it all. She kept making those choices that prohibited the path from ascending. She made one bad choice after another, failing at everything, accomplishing nothing, living life like a row of falling dominoes. Her world was crashing and burning but she didn't see what was happening.

There was once a girl who blamed all of her wrongs and problems on others, pointing fingers at her father and everyone around her. Playing the blame game, in her head, she yelled, "It is your fault that I am this way! It is your fault that my life is so grey!"

There was once a girl who was near the end. She didn't know if she would make it much longer, knowing the things she did, the drugs she mixed, and those times she lay there thinking it was her last. Lying with strangers, hoping they would be the one to do the deed for her, she was left in a hotel on drugs, hoping they would call it murder.

There once was a girl who wanted to give up. She wanted nothing but to see death's door. Knowing once she knocked upon it, that she would be free, giving her loved ones a chance to finally breathe.

Then, she saw a light. The light was so bright that even through only a crack, it lit up the room.

Today, there is a girl who found yoga. She stepped on the mat and got higher than the time she wrote her full name in cocaine and thought she touched the sky.

Today, there is a girl who wanted another chance. She looked over at the lives of others, the smiles they wore, the laughter they sang, and she wanted to feel that same thing.

Today, there is a girl who stopped pointing fingers away from herself and took fault for her mistakes. She found a new path and never looked back.

Today, there is a girl who creates moving art in human form. She enjoys feeling all of the sensations from the tingle in her toes while sitting in *janu c* pose to the amount of work it takes for her body to hold her up in a handstand, which gives the fly-so-high feeling when her feet touch the sky.

Today, there is a girl who has found gratitude for life. She gives thanks to the stars for the path that is provided. She smiles at wrongs and problems, knowing that they are lessons and guidance.

Today, there is a girl who replaced the hate with happiness. She smiles when her feet hit the mat and she even smiles when she crashes.

Today, there is a girl who decided to go against the grain of things. She believes in magic. She watches herself transform daily through this practice we call yoga, and it all started with asanas as simple as baby cobra.

Today, there is a girl who wants to make a difference. She lives to show the world what this magical practice can do, for it changed her life and she knows it can change yours, too.

Today, there is a girl who found her dharma, right here in a little town called Parma.

Today, this girl has dedicated herself to helping others by using this yoga practice to guide people toward helping themselves and one another.

Today, this girl uses her voice, as she knows your life and what you do is your choice.

The Stranger
Fiction by Nikki Martin

It was early. The sun had pressed its way up into the sky before she'd arrived at the beach, but Cara wasn't sure if it had been an hour or even two since that first peek of daylight over the rolling hills. The light was strange this morning. Mystical. There was a perpetual state of dusk, that pinkish hue of early evening light that had no place in the morning. She felt a lingering state of change that pulsed and flowed around her like a living, breathing thing.

She'd come this morning as she did every day in the summer months. Each morning she would dive into the sea, strong sure strokes carrying her out to those deep, familiar waters and then she would turn around and savor every stroke that carried her back to shore. She would return to the sand and practice yoga in the sun. As she rose and folded, stepped and stretched, she would let her breath reach in and out again almost as if she were still swimming. Swimming, she believed, was much like yoga, just a different kind of trying to get somewhere while landing right here in the moment.

She'd been doing both things as far back as she could remember. She'd always loved the water, the ocean especially, and growing up with a mother who taught yoga for a living had brought her to that practice at a very young age. There was a brief time when she had lost her way, and that practice of landing either on her mat or practicing on the beach when the weather was warm had stopped. But she found her way back, just when she needed to most.

While she stood on the beach now, the waves went from these loudly whispering giants to heavy, lazy things that could barely speak as they lay down at her feet in surrender. She watched a seal waltz with the waves, a lone paddle boarder grow tall as he or she neared the shore, birds dived for play or meals or pleasure. The ocean carried them all slowly, slowly towards her to be discovered.

And she thought to herself, *so this is what life is supposed to be, this slow and quiet unfolding piece by piece, detail by detail, of the world around me.*

And then she realized that she was not alone.

Cara didn't have to look to know that the boy, "the Stranger" had come again. She knew that he was standing still as a midnight moon, watching the ocean as she did, and yet seeing it in a way that she could not, not yet. He watched with eyes older than time, older than the sea and the stars and the moon. When she finally looked down at him, and the child who wasn't a child at all looked up at her and met her gaze, those eyes carried her back, back, and she remembered that she had looked into those eyes before, on the day her life had changed forever, though he hadn't been a boy then, had he?

***

Cara and her mother, Liz, had been heading home from the yoga studio where her mother taught five days a week. Cara drove as her mind chased a thought her mother had planted in her mind while she'd been in that final pose of rest and reward, savasana. Liz had guided them through a fiery and fierce vinyasa class, challenging sequences strung together with fluid movement. Liz loved to teach like that. Fire and water danced together to prompt a washed-clean feeling seventy-five to ninety minutes later.

Liz knew firsthand how powerful a practice like that could be. Throughout her life, she'd returned to that practice herself to be rid of the many demons that had first led her to yoga. Fire, the great consumer, could be used to burn away all kinds of negative thoughts and emotions, things you didn't need, things that held you back, things that weighed you down. There was no end to what you could offer that fire as long as you let it build and surrendered to it, and then you could use it, a different kind of cleansing than the flowing and fluid movement that followed and allowed you to catch your breath and cool the flames.

She'd moved them through fire and water over and over again, until that final extinguishing when they could rest. And that's when Liz would speak. Would lead them down roads she'd long ago travelled and then set them off on their own to find their way in those final minutes in savasana.

That particular night she'd said something that Cara could not escape, and so now she chased it down instead. Her mother had said that yoga, whether on your mat or out in the world, was the practice of knowing yourself. She'd said that stepping into this lifetime was like a great unraveling. That before this we were completely whole, and the true path of a lifetime was in knitting ourselves back together again and in finding our way back to that divine light, that great whole of creation and love, that unites all. She'd said our purpose was finding that true self, the one that had become a stranger to us the moment we were born. Liz had said we do this through practice, we do this by living with love and compassion, and we do this by answering the question: what do I have to offer the world that is mine alone to give?

So it was all of this that Cara was chasing when the drunk driver ran the red light and slammed into the passenger side of their car. Even in that moment that would feel like an eternity, that would slow down and stretch out between the sounds of tearing metal and breaking glass all around her, there wasn't enough time to make sense of what was happening or how her life was changing, irreversibly, with Cara powerless to do anything about it but scream.

Later, when there was only silence, before the sirens broke the eerie quiet and announced that help was coming, she lay gasping on the side of the road, pain streaking up her side to land in her chest, the taste of blood in her mouth and the smell of fire and other awful things in the air, she met "the Stranger" for the first time.

Cara had somehow gotten out of the burning car and was sprawled on the pavement and a beautiful old woman was cradling her head in her lap. She felt a pressing down on her chest as the woman, "the Stranger," stroked her blood-streaked hair and hummed under her breath.

Cara stayed calm and she believed she would be okay. When she met the Stranger's eyes, her head swam and her vision blurred. There were secrets and truths lurking within them that chilled her, things no person could know in the single leap that was a lifetime; and maybe no person was meant to. But for a moment, right before passing out, Cara swam into those depths, and for just a moment she was sure of her place in the intricately woven fabric of existence, and then everything went dark.

***

Cara looked at the empty bottle of prescription-strength sleeping pills in her hand and then let them tumble to the carpet. She'd swallowed every last pill and chased them each with a mouthful of vodka. She was too young, she thought, to think that this life did nothing but wound, and hurt and scar you. She was tired of working and waiting to heal. She was tired and she was broken. If only she could rest, could sleep and sleep, and wake up in another life. God, she hoped that's how it worked.

It had been two years since the day her mother had been taken from her in the car accident, and still the pain could tear her in two as if it happened only a moment ago. And in some ways it had, because Cara's life had stalled that day and hadn't moved forward since. She could still recall the sweet smell of her mother's hair after she'd washed it, the soft and firm touch she'd apply when giving an adjustment in yoga class. She could remember the sureness of her voice as she led a room full of people through a practice.

She remembered her mother's eyes, and that deep and honest longing to find her own way and to help others find theirs. Cara wasn't sure anymore if she held onto these things out of love or longing but they were with her just the same.

Cara slowly became aware of the Stranger standing in her bedroom. The realization of his presence reached through the fog of sleeping pills and vodka. He stood in the corner of her bedroom, watching.

He was monstrous in a way. Flesh, long ago charred, knit together in angry tangles and knots of red and pink skin and covering every inch of him. When she met the Stranger's eyes, she knew she would never be the same. Light and dark, day and night, eternities piled on top of one another, and a knowing so vast it stopped her breath in her throat. *We aren't meant to look into those kinds of depths are we*, she thought, remembering the hauntingly fathomless eyes of the beautiful old woman who'd cared for her on the night her mother had died, yet she could not look away.

As she lay on the floor, the room beginning to spin around her, unconsciousness beginning to tug at her edges, she swore she could smell the fire that had consumed the Stranger; and for just an instant she was transported fully back to the night when her entire life had changed. And when that smell hit her nostrils—imagined or real—that burning of things that were not meant to burn, Cara was propelled upward with revulsion and managed to get to the bathroom before being sick over and over again until she was sure she had been emptied out entirely. Then she lay down on the cold white floor and closed her eyes. She was certain as she drifted off into the darkness it was for the very last time and her final thought was that she wasn't ready to go; she'd been mistaken.

The next morning she woke in her bed. She had no clear memory of the night before or the Stranger in her room but something was different; she was different. It was summer and for the first time since the day her mother died, she rose and put on her swimsuit and headed to the beach. When she got there she dived into those familiar waters to let the ocean soothe her soul, and intuitively reached for the horizon again and let her breath and body lead her out to deeper waters until some instinct deep within told her to stop and turn around.

When she returned to the shore she practiced yoga on the sand for the first time in two years. Though her body was stiff and maybe not as open as it had once been, she remembered, and she began to find her way back to herself, slowly, back to that stranger waiting within to be discovered and known. For the first time since the world had ripped her mother's life away from hers, she felt hopeful; grateful for this tiny drop of a life in the vast ocean of existence. And she understood that to be a part of that ocean, that eternal ebb and flow, meant that we do not begin and end, we simply move in and out of lifetimes, each one like a wave upon the sea.

***

Cara let go of all of the remembering and looked down at the Stranger, the little boy who wasn't a boy at all, and she smiled. He had been coming to her since she'd found out she was sick, since she'd been told she only had a few months to live. That first day she'd seen him on a street corner staring at her intently as she stumbled home, shocked, breathless, unsure what to do exactly with being told her life would not be what she'd always thought, and expected, and hoped that it would. He'd never spoken in all the time he'd come to her, but he always seemed to arrive just when she was ready to give up hope, to give in, and somehow his presence would calm and quiet her. When she met his eyes she'd remember what she'd felt just a moment before a drunk driver had slammed into her car and ended her mother's life in an instant more than five years before: that it wasn't always easy...that beauty could be in the struggle...that her mother had taught with that fire that you had to be willing to suffer and burn through because in life, just as in yoga, the greatness was in being willing to both fight and surrender.

She stared out at the ocean, dusted with that strange pink light that had no place in the morning, and wondered if this pull towards the sea that was within her, within us all, was simply a longing for our beginnings, for that first place that we called home before we were chased up onto the land however-many millions of years ago. She had often wondered if that eternal being, the Sea, had somehow known all that we would become—the destruction, the hate, the forgetting of where we came from and the soul of ourselves—and had cast us out all those years ago.

And Cara had wondered if we could ever return, be forgiven in a way that would let us somehow go back. Could we find that truth again that we forfeit when we choose to leap into these short and beautifully painful lifetimes?

It was then that she heard the waves whispering: come home, come home, come home, as they crashed into the shore, and she knew that of course we could, and that she was ready. She went to take the Stranger's hand and realized the boy was gone. Some steps must be taken alone.

And so Cara walked into the waves and she was carried home, back into that cradle of love and light.

The Break
Fiction by Shana Thornton

She paces up the street and lights the cigarette quickly. Her legs are stiff and quick. The stroller glides along in front of her. The nine-month-old baby looks out, grasping the edge of the plastic tray in front of him, and leans forward. He doesn't want to blink for fear of missing a passing sight. The summer's hot air lifts the front of his hair, as his mother propels them forward with her easy glide. She lowers the cigarette and tries to hide it behind her thigh as she stretches a tight smile across her face at the other moms and kids who are at the playground. The baby waves his hands in the direction of the children. She steers with one hand along the sidewalk and passes by the playground. She hurries past the towering, mosaic-tiled dragon with its shiny and chipped body that children climb along. Some pieces of the dragon's tile look dingy, and others are colorful with bright hopes and the easy scrape of a child's leg and blood dripping down without a child's tears; maybe a wince escapes, but is hastily forgotten, in the face of the colorful, laughing dragon.

She remembers the years when she was a child, climbing along the dragon's back, and she feels sadness for how time passes, and why she's still on West End when she had wanted Central Park or Golden Gate. Lost in fantasies, she nearly collides with a telephone pole. A flyer advertises a new yoga studio that's opening around the corner. She wanted to try yoga last year, but it took thirty minutes to get to the nearest studio. She's annoyed when her cigarette goes out while she reads the yoga flyer.

The humidity thickens, and the clouds squat like a noxious prediction in the sky. She strolls faster along the sidewalk, but reaches for the lighter to re-light her cigarette anyway. She can't smoke in the apartment or the courtyard, and this is her "me" time. She needs these breaks. If she can get away with it, some days she smokes on the dragon, puffing from the tail if no children are around. The stress of becoming a mother, starting a new job, and living in an apartment surrounded by nosy neighbors has been anxiety-inducing. If she didn't smoke, she doesn't know how she would ease her tension some days.

She tells herself stories to feel better—that the dragon protects her, understanding the smoke, knowing the need to take the edge off. But, today, she keeps going. Most of her friends and co-workers don't know she smokes. Yesterday during her break, she saw a neighbor crossing the street toward her and quickly flapped her hands to wave away the smoke. Today, the additional humidity shuffles her feet forward, even though continuing exacerbates a feeling akin to smothering.

She inhales and pulls with her lips, cheeks, her lungs, puffing and pulling and yanking through the cigarette for a release that won't fall today. Nothing changes inside her body. It remains frustrated and pulses hotter and hotter.

She begins to jog and puff on the cigarette until tears of sweat puddle around her eyes and pour from her head and cheeks, running underneath her hair, her pants and shirt, her bra and panties. It's as if the presence of the dragon follows her, smoldering her neck and the backs of her legs. She pushes the stroller harder, trying to reach the crosswalk before the light changes, watching the tiny stream of smoke from her cigarette flow in a current along her arm, streaming behind her. She trips and nearly stumbles to the ground. This sends sparks of fear along her fingers and toes, throughout her body, as she tries to stay on her feet and the stroller lurches forward into the intersection.

Shock sends prickling waves along every joint and muscle of her body.

She sees the clouds, in a thunderhead above the intersection that curls into a dancing dragon body, as if laughing. She scrambles forward desperately. There's a sudden scream, jerk, and steer. The car horns and stares startle her shame up into tears, but she manages to grab the handle of the stroller and get back to the sidewalk somehow as it rocks back and forth as if it might topple over sideways. The baby cries in fearful, panicked gasps.

"It's okay," she says aloud, with accusation, to remind herself more than the baby. Her fingers claw around the handle and she straightens the stroller as she continues to walk, and everything sounds like waves, as her heartbeat pounds out the fear. Suddenly, she notices with a jolt that her other hand still holds the cigarette, and it has burned down so far that the heat begins to sting her fingers. Still, the baby cries with a little shrill gasp at the end of each breath. The final puff of cigarette smoke catches the wind and blows up into her face. She tries not to cry and drops the cigarette butt. She feels splashes of rain and, relieved, stops to adjust the stroller canopy so that the baby won't get wet. Just as abruptly as the rain and her relief, the baby stops crying and laughs when he sees her face. From beneath the canopy, his fat fingers stretch out to touch the raindrops.

When she turns the corner, the new yoga studio is in front of her. "Acceptance that we are always changing" is a slogan printed on the window. The door is propped open. She doesn't even think twice as she pushes the stroller through the entry.

How To Quit Yoga
Poetry by C.T. Kern

You do not give it up,
that mystery that makes you stand
powerful, breathe calmly, collapse
in acceptance at the end
of the best hour of your week.
No. It is something you can do alone.

Like church, AA, or rock concerts,
it is not the same alone,
those minutes stretching
on the cement patio, outside the slider
where your toddler spies you with joy
then sobs smearily against the glass
desperate and yowling like a rescue animal
unchosen. The cat climbs on your stomach
plows into your hair, your ears,
your dangling arms. The neighbor's diesel
idles in his driveway.

You go back to class.
You are used to eating dinner now
in the late afternoon, before bath time.
So you do not think of breath
but of chicken korma, of pizza,
of the smoothies you think you'll make before class
but don't. The relaxation at the end
still works, your limbs weighted
like buckwheat pillows.

You take up running. You can run when you want
in the fresh morning before work.
Running responds to effort—
you play "Born to Run" and
you make your feet go.
You run up the big hill until

bits of your lungs tear themselves
off. It is the kind of sport that makes you
spit, makes you fierce,
makes you have shin splints.

Back at yoga, you find your hamstrings
clenched with the all-American effort.
Your toddler begs to go with you,
shows you her down dog—palms flat,
diaper in the air,
but Mommy and Me is across the 605,
on a work night; it might as well be the moon.
Your toddler gets a cold, you get a cold.
Imagine you are taking a break.

Home Hive
Fiction by Shana Thornton

Mia walked through the gate, unlooping the rope before creating a small opening and passing through quickly, and then looping the rope to close the gate again. She shrugged at the gate, thinking it unnecessary to signify a separation when there wasn't one anymore. All this land belonged together and this was a barrier from long ago. The barriers were divisions of how the people felt set apart and needed to show a sign of their possessions. The same could not be said of their neighbors on the other side of the eighty-acre yoga sanctuary her mom and dad owned, and so they had left the fences and gates, the barred ditch lines, and borders of high, manicured shrubbery in place.

She ran across the field close to the first of the tall summer weeds and at the edge, she stopped and pulled a step stool from behind the tree where she had left it yesterday. She climbed up and gathered the mulberries from the lowest branches of the tree. She was determined to get them before the birds and deer, and she smiled at herself as she gently pulled a branch down to her hand and plucked the berries from it. Even though she was only eleven, Mia was adept and thoughtful about being helpful to her parents. She enjoyed learning to cook and blend teas. Her mom wanted the berries to make something wild and special for the clients. Her mom said that mulberries and tea brewed from mulberry leaves meant wild zest, and her mom needed that spirit right now for some new clients.

The sanctuary was a wellness retreat center, and Mia's parents helped people from all kinds of backgrounds to find their ideas of freedom. Shapeshifter Sanctuary was their life's work, and they said that meant helping others change shapes in body, mind, and soul.

Mia's great-grandparents, then her grandparents, long-ago ran a successful hotel with twenty bedrooms, one of which was a Presidential suite, in this once-popular railway town, known for its healing spring and river waters. Several U.S. Presidents from the early 20th century visited, and the hotel accommodated all of them. Mia's dad had donated half of his inheritance to create Shapeshifter Sanctuary.

After she filled the bottom of a plastic bucket with berries and covered them with fresh leaves, Mia walked back toward the hotel. On the way, she noticed a long stick in the grass. She picked it up. "My wand," she said to the forest, as if saying those words would take away her apprehension to explore the woods. She heard something rustle the leaves, and she squatted to get a closer look.

The flash of golden flickered among the stinging nettle and forest undergrowth of vines and other invasive plants, as some people thought of them. She thought about the plants often and what her mom wanted to do with them and to the forest. Mom clapped her hands together in joy when she talked about the forest and what it had to offer. "We'll put some beehives out here. This is our sweet spot to make the world a better place, and we'll make it even sweeter."

While she thought about her mom's plans, a fox dashed onto the trail quickly, hopping through an old wooden fence, and disappearing into the fields of wildflowers. She hurried along the path until it suddenly turned from a grassy field bordered by wildflowers to a rock-lined, pine needle-covered, darkened forest trail under the evergreens. She shivered but there was a stillness that comforted her. A big rock appeared in the distance. She stopped abruptly when the fox circled in front of it, winding gracefully back and forth by itself, around nothing, through the air. It disappeared just as quickly over the little hill.

Mia ran on her tiptoes, now forgetting any caution or fear, allowing her toes to grip her curiosity and move her forward to chase the as-yet-unknown-to-her fox. When she finally came to the rock in the path, it was so large that she had to scramble up the side of it, trying not to slip and allowing her fingertips to find the little grooves and sharp edges that she had learned so well. She memorized those tiny ledges of its smooth surface where the dust carried on the winds had collected. She paused and took in deep breaths, quickly moving one of her hands free momentarily to push her sweaty hair behind her ear. And fearing that she'd lose her grip on the mulberry bucket, she quickly made a last awkward scramble to the top and anchored herself with a smile as she surveyed the path ahead. Straight ahead was a small orchard, a kitchen garden of plots, and the lawn circle where a group of women each stretched an arm up to the sky together, resembling skinny tree branches pointed toward the clouds.

The wind blew a sudden gust and Mia noticed a fluttering of colors billowing up behind the women. She squinted and thought they were laughing. She watched as the rainbow of fabrics flapped around the women's faces. The scarves were attached to their heads. When the women shifted into their next posture, swirling their hands from points to the sky and bending backwards, some of them touched all the way back to the ground behind them. Others reached their hands backward in a line, horizontal to the earth.

Mia's dad saw her at the same time and waved for her to come over to the class. She wanted to stay on top of the rock, to continue surveying the area from her favorite place. She was hoping to see the fox again, too, but it had disappeared once she ran toward the rock. Giving up the search with a shrug, she slid down the front of the rock. Some of the women looked at her while she crossed the field, but most continued to follow her dad's instructions. The women were seated on yoga mats of all different colors. By the time she reached the back steps to the hotel and placed her bucket in the shade, the women had formed a semi-circle like multi-colored petals on a flower. She realized that some of the bald heads belonged to both men and women as they shone in the sun, and the fuzzy, short hair of a few women pointed out in unruly spikes.

She could hear her dad now, telling the yoga students to breathe and stretch. He said, "Let's try to hold this stretch for five full breaths. With each exhale, try to stretch a little farther. Try to touch your toes, or try to grab your wrist if you can easily touch your toes. We all have different bodies, so the stretch will be different for everyone. Don't compare your flexibility to anyone else's."

Mia paused when the path changed into a sidewalk. She could see another class on the meditation platform of the hotel. The students used props and chairs to hold their bodies into postures. She could see the gleam of their wheelchairs and titanium body parts. The wounded warriors came to the sanctuary every day. Her mom's brown hands rested on the shoulders of a woman and gently pushed the woman forward so that her body made a straighter line. The woman smiled. Her mom's voice drifted on the wind, "I'm here to help you reach the stress," she said to everyone in her class. "Be patient in your balance and I'll be around to all of you." Her mom was a yoga therapist and a cook. Her mom said to the students, "If you feel restless, think of OM, even hum it if you need to. The sound vibration will anchor you." Her mom glanced up and waved as Mia stared at the class. Mia waved back.

She turned around and walked toward her dad's class of cancer survivors. Her dad's students were lying flat on their backs with their arms at their sides. Her dad tapped out a soft rhythm on a set of bongo drums with his fingertips. He waved and patted the ground as a signal for Mia to sit down beside him.

When her dad finished his instructions to the class for final relaxation, he gave Mia the rose oil infused with lavender flowers. Mia placed drops of the fragrance on small handkerchiefs and into the hands of the students who wanted aromatherapy after their yoga practice. Those who didn't want aromatherapy rolled up their mats. They watched Mia drop the oil on the handkerchiefs, and the students raise the cloths to their faces, their necks, and wipe it through their hair.

Everyone lingered. Mia blushed again as she finished her task and the students all stared and smiled. "Hi," she said.

"Hi, Mia."
"Namaste."
"Hello, beautiful one."
"Glad you're here today."

"Let's lead an OM meditation," Mia's dad said, suddenly. "For anyone who wants to stay. What do you say, Mia? Would you?"

Her face reddened with embarrassment, but the students who had already rolled their mats turned back and unrolled the mats. Every student sat expectantly looking at her. Nervously, she pulled her frizzy hair into a short ponytail so that it wouldn't tickle her face. Feeling collected, she sat cross-legged on the ground and placed the back of her hands on each knee so that her palms opened to the sky.

Mia enjoyed the OM meditation and she especially liked the way her voice made a rhythm and vibration. The OM felt as if an anchor was dropping from her body into the ground and sinking way down into the earth. When she described it to her mom, she had said, "That's a beautiful image," and Mia always wished she could come up with something beautiful for every meditation. She felt the vibration on her sides and imagined OM birds fluttering back and forth inside of her body—inside the cages of her bones.

Her dad sat in the circle beside her, one of his knees rested against hers, lightly touching. Mia closed her eyes. She began to vibrate with the OM sound, lightly and quietly at first. She heard the yogis from her dad's class join in softly until they hummed like little honeybees combing the fields of clover. Their fuzzy heads were like the bees' fuzzy legs. She deepened the sound to make it roll, and she envisioned them floating above the field, hovering in the sunlight, suspended in a constant OM vibration through their wings. The sunlight dripped honey in streams into their throats until everyone glowed in light.

At some point, while Mia was imagining the bees, the OMs shifted and began to take on a life of their own with different yogis. She noticed OMs beginning and ending at their own pace, with their own depth of vibration and intensity, and some sounded as if they were taking off for flowers on another horizon. They left and returned like bees going their own way and returning to the hive. There wasn't a queen or king with a louder OM than anyone else. Mia was indistinct from the group. Her dad's OM was merged into the group hum, but she knew he was there. Mia felt the meditation until she was simply breathing and then, she opened her eyes in the process. The circle had grown to include her mom's class. Mia could see all of them as one sweet, humming hive.

Who Am I?
Nonfiction by S. Teague

I am you. I am the person who gets stares from onlookers. I am the person who has been wounded. I am the person who has won and the person who has lost. I am the person who has cried for help and the person who did it all by herself. I am the person who can stand in a crowd and the person who has major social anxiety. I am the person who has loved and the person who has been heartbroken. I am the person who has loved me and the person who has hated herself. I am anarchy and order. I am monochrome, and I am color. I am complicated and simple. I am no drama and high maintenance. I am a person who is real with life and still tells herself little lies to cope. I am uncaged and fearful of true freedom. I am mindful and thoughtless. I am giving and selfish. I am the person who has been wrong and the person who has been right. I am the person who has been accepted and the person that doesn't fit the mold. I am the person who has been hurt and the person who did the damage. I am the geek and the jock. I am one of the saved and have fallen from grace. I am success, and I am failure. I am a person willing to try and a person who is tired of trying. I am forgiving, but I am also a person with grudges. I am a moon child and a soul of the sun. I am a person who is relatable, but I am the person no one understands. I am in tune with hurt. I am in tune with glee. I am a bleeding heart, and I believe in personal power. I can feel your hurt, and I can rejoice in your recovery. I am an addict, but I have always been clean. I have walked the mile, and I have seen your shoes on my journey. I am all of you. We are one.

ABOUT THE CONTRIBUTORS

S. TEAGUE: S. Teague selected the contributors for *BreatheYourOMBalance* Volume One. She is the co-author of *Seasons of Balance: On Creativity and Mindfulness* (Thorncraft, 2016). From S. Teague: "As a recovering approval addict, I turned to what seemed to be my place in this world and allowed myself to become self-aware by beginning a personal yoga journey in 2014. My inner artist and creator emerged. Through photography and prose, I came home to who I was always meant to be—an artist. As I took on many shapes and forms artistically, my approval obsession silenced while my art grew. I began to breathe in this new life for myself. All I needed was a little salt." Find her on Instagram as @saltlifepirateprincess.

KARISSA BECKER: "I am that I am—I am a Mamasté (at home) With Her Little Oms, my sweet Starseeds are five and seven years old, and I have been married to the love of my life for eight years now. We move often and live fearlessly, and I am grateful for the IG platform where I can share my practice with you all from wherever we are in the world! May my stories inspire you as you delve deeper into your own journey. Sat Nam, the truth is within you." Find her on Instagram as @thegivingmom.

AMY RENEE BELL spent her growing up years in Saudi Arabia, then later in Montana. She greatly enjoys diversity of peoples and cultures and has traveled to many different places around the world throughout her life, which has shaped her perspective, her love of others, and her affection for nature and being outdoors. As a trained biology teacher, she loves instilling a love of science and nature to her students. Yoga is also an important part of her life, as well as training for triathlons and marathon swims. She does this while being a wife and mother of three, living near Salt Lake City, Utah. She has been practicing yoga for fifteen years and loves where the journey has taken her, both with things that apply specifically to fitness and on a much deeper emotional level as well. Find Amy on Instagram as @ufi_yoga

JACQUITTA BOONE is a beginner yogi and current ECU student. She is working towards her MBA with a concentration in Project Management. She began her yoga practice at home in December 2014. Since then, she is learning the true meaning of self-worth, self-love, and perseverance. Her love of yoga has progressed and led her to pursue her 200 hr. Yoga Teacher Training Certification in Greenville, NC, in the fall of 2016. She is a body positive advocate who also promotes self love. She hopes to share more of her love of yoga through her Blog, This Curvi Yogi (http://thiscurviyogi.com). Find her on Instagram as @Eyes_of_Sunshine.

ARIEL BOWLIN was born and raised in the Puget Sound area. She graduated from Western Washington University with a Bachelor's in Spanish and worked as a contract interpreter for the State of Washington for several years. She also taught Spanish Conversation at Everett Community College. Chronic injuries led her to practice and teach Yoga and Pilates. She now lives and teaches in Tucson where she loves to hike, read and practice Yoga in the park. She is a breast cancer survivor. Find Ariel on Instagram as @arielbowlin.

SARAH CUNNINGHAM is a Licensed Clinical Social Worker with eleven years of experience working alongside children, teens, and adults in an effort to empower and support the attainment of their individualized, therapeutic goals. For the past three years Sarah has been teaching yoga to both adults and children at her therapeutic yoga studio, Whole Life Wellness Studio, as well as in school systems across the greater Chicago area. She uses her clinical experience to inspire her yoga classes, leading to what her students have come to refer as "Sarahpy". Driven by passion about the healing properties of food, Sarah offers individual and group support for clients looking to learn more about how dietary changes can support their therapeutic goals. Read her blogs and writings on her website: http://www.sarahcunningham.com.

Sarah's writings are inspired by her personal and professional experiences, including world travel, that have informed her unique combination of both the western and eastern healing approaches of psychotherapy, yoga, and nutrition. You can follow her posts via Instagram @sarahcwellness and on the Whole Life Wellness Studio Website at www.wholelife-studio.com

Finally, Sarah would be delighted to gain you as a friend on Facebook at https://www.facebook.com/sarahcunninghamwellness.

SUMMER BREEZE FLOWERS: "California native, mother to two amazing little ones who have helped on my journey to finding my breath. Currently teaching yoga and loving it. Life is always presenting us with moments trying to take our breath away, so we must always look for it!" Find her on Instagram as @atimeforflowers.

JESSICA GIBBS is a pediatric physical therapist and began a daily yoga practice in December 2013. Her yoga journey has changed her life, both on and off the mat. She shares her love of yoga with everyone she meets and hopes to inspire others to practice kindness and love on a daily basis. Jessica resides in Atlanta, Georgia with her dog, Mate. Find her on Instagram as @gibby_smalls.

LILY GOMEZ: "Mom of three boys.
Yoga teacher.
Forever learning.
Smiling is my favorite asana." Find her on Instagram as @mymatisyourmat.

BARBARA LEE GRAY is an English Instructor at Austin Peay State University in Clarksville, Tennessee. She plays percussion, drums and other instruments. She produces her own music, which includes funk pop, rock and meditative pieces that include gong recordings. She acquired her first gong in the winter of 2012, when she started playing gong meditations for a variety of groups and in various situations.

DEB HARANO has lived in Colorado Springs since 1992, when she reunited with her high school sweetheart. They blended their young families together and created a new home. Deb has a strong interest in maintaining a daily yoga practice, healthy lifestyle and prefers natural healthcare practices. She has held many jobs, but is currently focused on teaching yoga, continuing her studies and planning to complete her advanced teacher training in 2016. She enjoys being a grandparent and dabbling in amateur photography. Deb also enriches her personal asana practice through social media, particularly through Instagram, as

@ColoradoYogaLady Her Website: http://www.dimensionsyoga.com

RUBY HERNANDEZ is a personal coach, yoga instructor, and psychotherapist. Her passion is in empowering people to heal from past trauma, gain deep presence for themselves, and find comfort and joy in the divine body they live in. Ruby helps people up-level their health+wellbeing and connect to their own 'inner glow' via yoga/mindfulness meditation, EFT tapping, and EcoTherapy adventures in nature. She also facilitates mind/body retreats in Costa Rica. Visit her website at http://www.LotusGlow.com Find her on Instagram as @Inner_Lotus_Glow.

Crystal-collecting, mystical mama, **BRITTANY HOOGENBOOM**, is fueled by the fire of love. She once was lost but now is found, thanks to yoga. She is a physical therapist assistant, yoga teacher, reiki master, metaphysical adept in training, and is earning a Bachelor's degree in alternative medicine—she literally never stops. Chasing her dharma to help the mother of the stars to heal the lives of human beings, she is empowered by gratitude. Find her on Instagram as @ladiboomyogini.

C.T. KERN lives near Los Angeles. Her work has been published in *The Florida Review, Image, Passages North,* and other journals. She has served as fiction editor of *The Cream City Review* and faculty advisor for *The West Wind* literary magazine.

STEPHANIE LASHER has been making magic and mischief since 1983. A true creative spirit and lifelong movement artist, she lives, writes, dances, and plays yoga in Maine with her loving husband and Samoyed pup, Loki. Share in the nonsense on Instagram with her as @freedivegirl.

LOIS McAFFREY LOPEZ attended Bryn Mawr College as a McBride scholar (program for women of non-traditional age), receiving a degree in Cultural Anthropology in 2003. In her younger life, she founded a specialized construction company, which she owned and managed for twenty years. After receiving the degree from Bryn Mawr, she spent a number of years working with non-profit agencies as well as finding adventure by sailing the Intercoastal Waterway and Caribbean seas with her husband. Her educational background, prior business experience, and time spent observing have given her a unique perspective from which to approach her view of the world and it is clearly evident in her writing. She received a Master's Degree in Creative writing from Wilkes College in 2013.

NIKKI MARTIN is a yoga teacher and writer living on the east coast of Canada with her partner, Paul, and a very strange cat named Girlie. They live on an acre of land in a quiet neighborhood just ten minutes from the ocean. In the summers, they grow as much of their own food as they can as well as keep honeybees. Both are passionate about doing what they can to help the environment, and for that reason, among others, Nikki is also a vegan.

Her love of stories, both reading and creating them, started very young when she realized they could be both escape and salvation for a shy, sensitive and awkward kid who always felt a little bit out of place, despite having friends and being very social. She drafted her first novel in grade nine and her first feature length screenplay not long after that, and has written many of both genres since. She hopes to sell some of her work in the coming years and continue to share her passion for yoga while teaching and travelling.

Nikki is an avid reader, a daydreamer, a movie lover, a sunset chaser, a love and laughter spreader, a beach walker, a storyteller, and an ocean soul.

SELWA MITCHELL was diagnosed at age three with the fatal, genetic disease Cystic Fibrosis. As she watched her mother fall to her knees from the doctors' news that her baby girl was not expected to live past seven years of age, Selwa Mitchell's fight began right then and there in that cold hospital room. Now at age 38, Selwa's mental and physical scars have found their home in her soul creating a fighter who won't take hearing, "You can't" from others lightly. Wife, mother to two healthy children, accountant and 200hr registered yoga teacher (RYT), Selwa lives the life she wants despite often being told that the odds are against her—something that just fuels her soul. On June 25th, 2016, at four am, Selwa's lungs took their last fighting breath for her. The journey up until her lungs last breath tested every ounce of Selwa's faith and mental strength. She fights hard despite the struggle, despite the difficulty because she knows every breath was worth the fight that led to knowledge and appreciation. To be alive is an understood blessing when each day has no guarantee. Uniquely, in her struggle, Selwa found a gift that bought her time and eased her pain. It is a gift that rejuvenated a tired soul and gave her power—Selwa found the gift of yoga. Follow her on Instagram as @selwayoga.

Ever since she started classes with her mum when she was 16, yoga has been a regular part of **LAURA SWAN POLLARD'S** life. She trained to become a yoga teacher in her home town of Brighton, UK and has been teaching for the past year. Laura's classes are grounded in acceptance and patience—there's no judgment, no force, no pressure. For her, yoga is all about taking time out for self and physical and mental health. Find her on Instagram as @swan_yoga.

TRACY M.G. RIGGS: Purveyor of all things adventuresome, wife, dog owner, visual artist, yoga instructor, daydream believer, Egyptian in a former life, soul gypsy. Find her on Instagram as @zephyra.yoga.

JASMIN SERINA is a registered nurse living in Tucson, Arizona. She was born and educated in the Philippines. She earned her Bachelor's degree in Business Administration, major Accounting, in her late teens. She finished her Bachelor's degree in Nursing soon afterward. Jaz migrated to the USA to pursue her nursing career. She had spent time as a health care volunteer in Cambodia and Philippines. She recently came back from Peru where she was a conservation volunteer. Her budding yoga journey has been inspired by her instructors, family and friends. Find her on Instagram as @jazser4.

KATIE SCHROEDER is a yoga practitioner, teacher, and ostomate who found healing inside and out through her dedication to yoga and trusting her gut, even though she had hers removed. Her raw honesty about her chronic illness and ileostomy has inspired many. She has helped several ostomates navigate the unknown territory of learning to thrive with an ostomy, and she spreads awareness about the unique condition that led to hers through print and social media. Katie is incredibly grateful for her yoga practice which helped her survive until having her life-saving surgeries. Yoga inspired her to love life with her ostomy. Her website: http://www.stomiyogi.com

LAURA ROSE SCHWARTZ is an Experienced Registered Yoga Teacher with Yoga Alliance (E-RYT 200), and a Balance Body-trained pilates instructor. She studied Interdisciplinary Yoga at the Nosara Yoga Institute in Costa Rica—an internationally-recognized yoga teacher training program. Laura focuses her yoga classes on vinyasa flow, which is full of movement and unique sequencing. She also teaches invigorating and challenging pilates and barre classes, utilizing isometric movements and creativity sequencing. Her classes are a balance of strengthening flow and breath—designed to be challenging, rewarding, and fun for all levels. Laura's background in science and anatomy allows her to utilize her knowledge of the body's physiology as she assists and informs her students. Laura also likes to share her love of music, and tries to ensure that her playlists are just as engaging as her techniques. An attorney in her previous life, Laura now spends her days much more happily teaching yoga, barre, and pilates full-time, and is also the Director of the studio where she teaches. Find her on Instagram as @lauraroseyoga.

LESLIE STORMS is a yoga teacher, registered nurse, marriage and family therapist, a published author, and a social media consultant, who has devoted herself to awakening. Her immense affinity for healing, learning, and transforming has led her to what can only be discovered by taking a look within. She holds a Bachelor's degree in Nursing and worked as an operating room nurse for over ten years. She completed her Master's degree in Marriage and Family Therapy, and upon graduation, she launched a successful solo practice. After five years, she had an epiphany—her heart was being called to expand. She had fallen in love with yoga, and its ability to transform oneself. She has taught and practiced various methods of yoga for over thirteen years. For the past three years, she has devoted herself to the six-day-a-week practice of the ashtanga yoga method. The ashtanga method offers the practitioner a self practice which allows for in depth self-study. She is grateful to the countless healers who have shared their experience and knowledge with her. Currently, she has graciously dedicated this life to connecting with stillness daily. She studies the teachings of Adyashanti and Paramahansa Yogananda. She has been honored with the acceptance of attending one of Adyashanti's highly sought-after silent retreats this winter. She longs to share her love of yoga, meditation, creative photography, and the ultimate, which to her is bravely committing to the journey of delving inside. Find her on Instagram as @lesliestorms.

CLARISSA MAE THOMPSON is a 200-hour registered yoga teacher (RYT), and she completed her training in Rock Island, IL, at

Tapas Yoga Shala with Evan and Kelly Harris in May 2014. She maintains a dedicated ashtanga practice and spent time in Mysore, India in December 2015, studying at the KPJ Ashtanga Yoga Institute with Sharath Jois. She has also spent time with a variety of knowledgeable teachers. These experiences feed her desire for knowledge and influence her class flows. Clarissa teaches regular classes at studios and online. She is also an avid blogger, writing about her personal experiences and life on and off the mat. Visit her Instagram account @clarissa_mae_

Her website: http://www.clarissamae.com

REGAN WARNER is an American living in the UK for the past eight years. She's a mummy, a wife, a baker, a creative director and a yogi. She started practicing in Detroit in 2001, and she took her registered yoga teacher training (200-RYT) in New York in 2007. She loves marrying her two passions together: design and yoga. This is evident on her Instagram account, @reganwarner, as she's continually hosting challenges with eye-catching graphics. Her goal is to always be honest and authentic with the ethos; work hard, stay humble. Find her on social media. Her website is http://reganwarner.com, and her Instagram is https://instagram.com/reganwarner.

BONNIE WEEKS loves a challenge. Her garage is her home studio for a weight-throwing or plyometric workout as well as the space she practices yoga. If there's something that seems hard, she's not afraid of it. She professes always moving forward and is a trainer and teacher who wants students to come away feeling powerful, important, and loved. She thrives on connecting movement with soul, the sacred in you. Bonnie is from Oregon where she lives with her husband, three children, and the beautiful, green Earth. Find her on Instagram at https://www.instagram.com/carrot_bowl_bonnie/ And, on her Website: http://carrotbowl.com.

CHELSEA WISE: "For twenty years, I have had the honor of working and studying with a diverse array of teachers, from shamans to midwives. My work as a yoga teacher, healer and artist is a process of connecting and returning. It is the journey of making the unknown, known. It is the acknowledgment that everything is alive and the conversation that is longing to be heard. It is the accessing of a profound power in the innate intelligence within us and all around us."

Find Chelsea Wise online via her photography on Instagram as @astheheronflies. Her Yoga practice on Instagram @chelsea_wise_ Her website: http://www.chelseawise.ca/

ARIELLE WITT-FOREMAN is mother to three-year-old Belle and a student of Entertainment Business at Full Sail University. She currently resides in North Carolina and enjoys spending time with Belle on the beach, practicing yoga, reading, writing and occasionally attending concerts. Find her on Instagram as @the_amazing_arielle.

ABOUT THE SERIES EDITORS

KITTY MADDEN is Thorncraft Publishing's Senior Editor. She not only edits every book multiple times as a line and content editor, but she also helps with strategy and overall planning for the publishing company. Kitty is known as Thorncraft's literary midwife, bringing out the best writing from all of our authors. Kitty was once a professional proofreader, nanny, and substitute teacher. She is currently a Reiki Master, practicing in Clarksville, TN.

SHANA THORNTON is the owner of Thorncraft Publishing, an independent publisher of literature written by women. She created the BreatheYourOMBalance brand and book concepts. Writing is her passion, and she is the author of two novels, *Poke Sallet Queen and the Family Medicine Wheel* (2015) and *Multiple Exposure* (2012). She is the co-author of the nonfiction self-help book, *Seasons of Balance: On Creativity and Mindfulness* (2016). Shana earned an M.A. in English from Austin Peay State University. She was the Editor-in-Chief of Her Circle Ezine, an online women's magazine featuring authors, artists, and activists. To read Shana's interviews with women authors and activists, visit Her Circle Ezine at www.hercircleezine.com
To read more of her nonfiction, visit her blog at www.shanathornton.com
Follow her on Twitter @shanathornton and find her on Instagram as @shana_trailbalance

BOOKS BY THORNCRAFT PUBLISHING

Nonfiction

BreatheYourOMBalance: Writings about Yoga by Women, Volume One, Selected and introduced by S. Teague (October 2016). A collection of poetry, fiction, and nonfiction that focuses on breath and balance, this volume celebrates the life-changing practice of yoga. Thirty contributors share their experiences in this first collection.
ISBN-13: 978-0-9979687-0-5
Library of Congress Control Number: 2016953726

Seasons of Balance: On Creativity & Mindfulness by S. Teague and Shana Thornton (March 2016). Teague and Thornton co-write a book about creativity, meditations, affirmations, expressions of gratitude and mindfulness to help you through the seasons of life. Use this book as a creativity journal to inspire you and to prompt artistic creations.
ISBN-13: 978-0-9857947-9-8
Library of Congress Control Number: 2016931608

Fiction

Talking Underwater by Melissa Corliss DeLorenzo (August 2015). Authors have declared that this novel is a "literary gift" and that "book clubs will love this." Cattail, the adored beach near her coastal New England home, is Amy's place of refuge. When a mistake there ends tragically, almost destroying everything that Amy holds as sacred, she doesn't know how she'll continue, nor mend the rift with her sister that results. *Talking Underwater* explores the balance between the elation of family summers at the ocean and the ways we navigate unbearable heartache to find new ways of being. ISBN-13: 978-0-9857947-6-7
Library of Congress Control Number: 2015938787

Poke Sallet Queen & the Family Medicine Wheel by Shana Thornton (March 2015). When narrator Robin Ballard takes a writing course in college, she goes searching for her homeless father and wanders into the secret lives of her ancestors and relatives. Set in Nashville and the surrounding communities, this novel offers a glimpse into the superstitions and changes of a middle Tennessee family.
ISBN-13: 978-0-9857947-5-0 LCCN: 2015901106

The Mosquito Hours by Melissa Corliss DeLorenzo (April 2014). One turning-point summer places the grandmother, aunt, daughter, granddaughters, and great-grandchildren in the same home. An OnPoint Radio suggestion as Best Summer Reads 2014, *The Mosquito Hours* is a multi-generational story about how the women in a family attempt to keep secrets about their desires, spirituality, and motherhood. ISBN-13: 978-0-9857947-2-9
Library of Congress Control Number: 2013957635

Grace Among the Leavings by Beverly Fisher (August 2013). Hailed by award-winning author Barry Kitterman as "a deeply moving story, one not given to easy resolution," this historical novella is a child's perspective of the Civil War. Playwrights Kari Catton and Dennis Darling adapted the book for the stage. Visit thorncraftpublishing.com for upcoming performances. ISBN-13: 978-0-9857947-3-6
Library of Congress Control Number: 2013938285

Multiple Exposure by Shana Thornton (August 2012). The "war on terror" has captured the lives of the U.S. military and their families for over ten years, and Ellen Masters' husband has been repeatedly deployed. In the process, she shares her desires to connect with people and to discover her own strength by training for a marathon. ISBN-13: 978-0-615-65508-6
Library of Congress Control Number: 2012941646

Forthcoming
BreatheYourOMBalance: Writings about Yoga & Healing, Volume Two.
The second volume of writings about yoga will focus on the healing aspect of the yoga practice. This book is being created in connection with Yoga Mat studio in Clarksville, TN, through a series of writing and yoga workshops.

For information about authors, books, upcoming reading events, new titles, and more, visit http://www.thorncraftpublishing.com

Like Thorncraft Publishing on Facebook. Find Thorncraft Publishing on Twitter as @ThorncraftBooks and on Instagram as @thorncraftpublishing